RAISING EMOTIONALLY INTELLIGENT CHILDREN

RENE ROBINSON

Copyright © 2021 by Rene Robinson

Paperback: 978-1-63767-580-9
eBook: 978-1-63767-581-6
Hardcover: 978-1-63767-612-7
Library of Congress Control Number: 2021922200

All rights reserved. No part of this publication may be reproduced, distributed, or transmitted in any form or by any electronic or mechanical means, without the prior written permission of the publisher, except in the case of brief quotations embodied in critical reviews and certain other noncommercial uses permitted by copyright law.

This is a work of nonfiction.

Ordering Information:

BookTrail Agency
8838 Sleepy Hollow Rd.
Kansas City, MO 64114

Printed in the United States of America

DEDICATION

To the children in my life.

I have always felt very privileged to have children in my care – little people who learned to trust me and to give me their love.

My fundamental belief was that, as a parent, teacher, grandparent or counsellor, I had the power to provide the BEST learning experience I could.

F or me, my work has been all about nurturing, loving and providing the children in my care with the greatest opportunities for growth and learning, all in a safe and secure environment.

Thank you to all who have been on this journey with me. It has been a fantastic experience.

CONTENTS

Chapter 1: How My Story Began 1
Chapter 2: Helping Your Child Develop
            Emotional Intelligence 23
Chapter 3: In My Classroom 33
Chapter 4: I'm a Carer – How Can I Help
            the Child in My Life? 42
Chapter 5: Building Trust in Children................................. 54
Chapter 6: Finding Your Centre 64
Chapter 7: Dealing With Toxic Shame................................. 86
Chapter 8: How to Show a Child They are Truly Loved 112
Chapter 9: Abuse 125
Chapter 10: Heart Truth 141
Chapter 11: Resilience 150
Chapter 12: Ways Children Learn About Life 165

Acknowledgements 176
About the Author 179
Endnotes 181

> "Children are the flowers of the earth."
>
> MAO TSE TUNG

CHAPTER 1

How My Story Began

My journey to become an educator and champion of children was not something I planned. Rather, this was a career that found me, at a time in my life when I was a single mother in conservative country Victoria, facing an uncertain future.

Over fifty years on, and having played an active role in guiding my own five beautiful grandchildren, I look back on all the children I have nurtured along the way with a great sense of pride and satisfaction. As well as teaching literacy and numeracy, the role I played in helping build the characters and emotional resilience of the young souls entrusted to me, became my life's work.

Even though my teaching days are over, my passion for this work continues. My hope in telling my story is that I am able to pass on to all carers of children, some of the invaluable lessons I've learnt along the way — about guiding children towards emotional wellness and strength, so they grow into healthy adults.

Please bear with me as you read this. I will use my own story, my sons' story, the stories of the children I have taught, as well as the story of my granddaughters, who I raised from infants — with their permission of course.

Through these stories, I will explain how emotions control our lives, influencing the very way we live.

I have made a decision not to name the people I describe in my book. If you can relate to any of these stories, just feel glad you have helped me learn and that my gratitude for the role you have played in my life is deep and sincere.

There is no blame intended in any of this book. I truly know that the experiences I've had in my life are all based on love and support. These were all lessons I chose to come and learn in this life and I am truly grateful for the people who have fulfilled these roles.

This book is very special to me. It felt as if it was channelled to me one morning as the words just seemed to flow. The day before we had been watching televised reports about the devastation caused by the Boxing Day Tsunami of 2004. My two granddaughters, Dakota, six and Summer, five, were with me, together with a young couple visiting with their two young children. There were so many questions as we watched the story unfold. As adults, we talked about how it was so important that children be encouraged to feel their emotions so they're able to understand more about themselves.

The following morning, I found an exercise book and the words just poured out. All of the work I had been doing myself and with my granddaughters around emotional intelligence, just seemed to be waiting for me to put it all down on paper. I had such a deep belief that children must be shown how to understand the emotions that flow through them so freely and be able to use this knowledge with confidence and ease.

It only took a few days to put it all down, and once finished, I put it away in a drawer. It took many years before I had the courage to present it to a publisher.

This is my story.

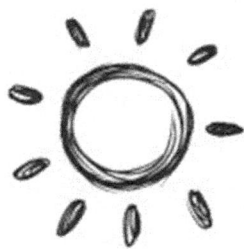

THE BEST LAID PLANS

After finishing school, I attended what was then known as Geelong Teachers' College and completed a two-year teacher training course. I married at the age of twenty-four, had three sons and left work to raise them. When the boys were around the ages of six, four and fifteen months old, my husband and I bought a seven-year lease on the Beech Forest Hotel Motel. My husband had become involved in managing hotels and he thought this would be good for us as a family. We tried very hard and for the first year we managed. However, the job of running a business like this doesn't give you much time for family life and ultimately, we lost everything we had, including our marriage.

I left Beech Forest and took the boys to Ballarat, to live as a single mum. My husband returned to his early home in Sydney.

At this stage the boys were nine, seven and four and we had no car, so it was very lonely and hard for me on my own.

I also realised that, with my marriage over, it would be up to me to support my three sons, so this was the beginning of my journey into the world of children's education.

Whilst we were living in Beech Forest, I had already begun off-campus studies for a Bachelor of Education/School Librarianship, and during our first year in Ballarat I completed enough units to qualify as a teacher/librarian. The second year I began work as a cataloguing librarian at Aquinas, the Ballarat campus of the Catholic Teacher Training University. I loved this work, but it was a stretch on my own, with three little boys, all at school.

In 1981, I applied to return to the Victorian Education Department as a teacher/librarian and gained a position at Portland South Primary School, where I taught for three years. As an added bonus, the boys and I were able to live in a school department house which gave us the security we needed. Studying was still a big part of my life because I wanted to achieve higher qualifications to be able to provide the life I wanted for my sons.

Even though the boys and I spent four happy years in Portland, I realised during this period, I was struggling emotionally and not dealing with my own feelings. Interestingly, I was aware of this in my boys and I encouraged them to deal with their own feelings – "Throw rocks at the back fence to get rid of your anger," I used to tell them.

During this time, I began studying again, off-campus, through Deakin University in Geelong. I completed four level three, and four level four units, mostly in the area of education. I was successful for a year, but it then became too difficult to keep up with the demands of study and the responsibility of raising my three boys on my own. So, in 1985, I agreed to a friend's offer to support me, so I could have a year off without pay to finish my course. As I was a student and a single parent, I was eligible for a certain amount of government assistance. I was also able to continue paying into my superannuation and I had the security of knowing there was a job waiting for me. Over this period, I completed enough units to be awarded a Bachelor of Education, through Deakin University's off-campus program. With this new qualification, I was now able to climb the career ladder in the education department.

I returned to work, confident the study I had completed would enable me to follow my ambition to help develop the school curriculum and perhaps become vice-principal if the opportunity arose. I ultimately did realise this dream when I became teacher-in-charge of a small rural school — just outside Horsham, in the north west of Victoria.

When my son Luke needed to repeat year nine, as he was considered too immature to go into year ten, I had no other option but to move the boys to Warrnambool Secondary School, where fortunately Luke thrived.

For the next four years the boys and I called Port Fairy home. We lived in two houses while we were there and this small community provided safety, as well as security for a single mum and her sons. During that time the boys took the school bus to Warrnambool, while I drove fifty kilometres in the opposite direction to Narrawong Primary School, where I was teaching at the time.

In 1989, I finished up at Narrawong Primary School and found a position at Koroit Primary School, so our lives changed once again.

During this time, I met a musician called Baz, who played brilliant guitar and lived in Wartook, a small town near Horsham. I fell in love with Baz and many weekends were spent on the road, travelling between our two houses in Port Fairy and Wartook.

Baz and I married in 1990, at the Kirks Reservoir Park in Ballarat and the boys and I moved to Baz's house in Wartook where I was able to transfer my teaching.

When I met and married Baz, he was bringing up his own two teenage daughters which meant between us we had five teenagers, aged thirteen to nineteen, and it was tough!

I was also missing the ocean. After four years living on the coast, in Port Fairy, no one warned me just how hard it would be to leave it behind, nor how much I would miss my oldest son, Luke, after he left home at the age of nineteen to attend TAFE in Geelong.

Although there was a deep love between Baz and me which brought happiness, managing teenagers with all their issues, travelling fifty kilometres to Horsham every day, the heat, and Baz's problem with alcohol, all proved too much, so, in 1998 I left the marriage. As I write this, I'm aware my own personality may have played a part in the failure of my relationships with men. The deep emotional pain I experienced from the teasing I suffered at the hands of my older brother taught me to seek out relationships with men where I felt stronger – men I could feel intellectually superior to and who I could really live without. I met beautiful men who were brilliantly creative, yet they were like my father and not able to 'put me in my place' when perhaps I needed to be. I remember saying to Baz that I needed a strong man who "could keep me down" and he was honest enough to say that this was not his way.

I think, because of my personality I became somewhat of a bully, something I learned with shame as I started working on my own personal development. I was intolerant of people who could not or would not stand up to me which was not a nice quality to have. I have since learnt much about myself over the years and I continue to learn so much more when listening and feeling the emotion, rather than allowing the anger to hide it all.

Looking back on this period, I was very angry and found this anger was escalating.

I lived with constant headaches – I would wake up in the morning with one, suffer throughout the day, go to bed with a headache and they would wake me in the middle of the night. They ranged from bad to unbearable, seriously affecting my moods. I was probably also going through menopause at the time which only made things worse. The only place I found I wasn't angry was with my class of children. I think that's because I found it easy to be my real self in their presence.

One morning, during this period, I woke up and the headache pain was so bad that I was unable to lift my head from the pillow. I went to see the doctor who told me there was nothing physically wrong with me and referred me to a spiritual healer who offered a class in personal development and self-awareness.

I attended this class and it helped me understand that I had buried my emotions and used anger as a shield, suppressing my feelings as a result. The effort required to internalise this anger had forced my body to physically react in this way, resulting in the blinding headaches I was suffering.

This experience marked the beginning of my journey into the study of emotional intelligence. I travelled regularly to Melbourne and attended the many courses taught by Nicholas de Castella, a master life coach and founder of the Australian Breathwork College. Nicholas is also a quantum breathwork trainer and works with mature people, teaching them practical emotional skills to empower themselves emotionally. Through the training I received from Nicholas, I learnt to acknowledge and let go of the pain I carried.

At this stage, I was only working with and releasing one emotion, my anger, and the process was cathartic, as well as loud!

As the years passed, I experienced more emotional challenges. My marriage to Baz had deteriorated and the kids were leaving home, so school became my favourite place to be – my sanctuary. I worked in a small rural school with only thirty-eight students over a period of four years. This meant I had some of these children each year, for the time I was teaching there. As a result, these students and I had built up trust in each other and I genuinely loved them.

During the second year and into the third year of my time at this school, nine of these children experienced deaths in their families – including a stillborn sister, a father, a little dog who used to visit the class every day, an aunt, and a beloved nanna. I knew I needed to do something to help these children deal with their grief and I believed I could adapt what I was learning myself about emotional intelligence to help the children. I did so and with fantastic results.

There was one particular young family, with six children, who moved into our area from Queensland, following a tragedy. The family had been enjoying a picnic one day, near a river and cliff, when the father took the two boys rock climbing. The father fell, hit his head and landed in the river. The mother jumped into the river to pull him out but, sadly, he had drowned. Following the incident, the mother left Queensland and moved into our community so she could be near her own family, enrolling four of the children, two boys and two girls, into our school. Before the children joined the school, I talked with the other students about their story because I knew they were emotionally intelligent and would be able to support these children. Even though the children in my class worked hard and were well behaved, every recess and lunch time, they would go outside, get all of the balls from the sports shed, and kick them over the back fence, into the paddock beyond. When the bell rang, they would go collect them and put them back, then, next break the same thing would happen again. I would come to understand, later, that this was in fact a healthy and effective way for the children to release any pent-up feelings they may have been experiencing.

When the grandmother of two of the other students was diagnosed with cancer, the work I was doing with teaching practical emotional intelligence became even more important, it was very simple and very effective, as I will explain later in my book. On the day of the grandmother's funeral, the children were sitting on the floor and one little girl asked if we could go to the funeral, and I replied, "No, it's not our place".

She asked, "So what happens at a funeral?" Amazingly, the little girl from Queensland, whose dad had tragically died, said quietly, "Can I please tell them about my dad's funeral?" Together, with her brother, the children told the class what happens at a funeral. I then said to the little boy, "You were very angry when you came to our school, how do you feel now?" In a very serious voice, he replied, "I miss him every day, but the anger has gone." I knew then that emotional wellness techniques and skills could be easily taught to children.

PASSAGE TO CHINA

At the end of 1997, and at the age of fifty-five, I decided I would retire the following April. In the meantime, I took my long service leave and applied for a position teaching English in China and was successful.

I left Australia in early March 1998, leaving behind my alcoholic husband and drug addicted son. My granddaughter was born just before I left Australia so leaving home and travelling so far was not an easy decision, but I felt I had to save myself. This was not my first trip to China. I had long been interested in Eastern philosophies and practices, in particular yoga and tai chi, and in 1994 I attended the Beijing Sports University to learn a form called Dao Yin, returning again in 1996. Tai Chi became one of the greatest passions of my life from then on.

In 1998 I travelled to China to take up a position as a foreign expert at the Central South Forestry University, in Zhuzhou – a city in the eastern Hunan Province of China. It was a fascinating place to be and, whilst there, I made many dear friends who cared for me during my time there.

The Chinese culture is very different to western culture with few opportunities for emotional release. In fact, I believe these beautiful people are taught from an early age not to show emotions and that they have no place in Chinese society. Because of this, while I was living there, I felt I had to bottle my feelings up, so as soon as I returned to Australia in 1999, I attended the first workshop I could and began to let it all go. This was Nicholas De Castella's 'Inaugural Radical Breakthrough Weekend' and I was one of Nicholas' earliest students.

Following my experience in China, I decided my chosen path was travelling to other countries and teaching English and started planning my next trip.

However, in 1999, fate stepped in and my plans changed. I took on the care of my two infant granddaughters, who were six weeks and eighteen months old when they came to live with me.

For three weeks, I had the responsibility for these tiny, precious girls, before they were placed in a foster home as authorities tried, unsuccessfully, to reunite their family. After many months of work, involving social workers and various government agencies, it was all in vain and the children were unable to return to their parents.

In March, 2000, my world totally and permanently changed when I became the prime carer of my granddaughters – who, at two-years and ten months old, were too young to understand what had happened to their lives. Their father, sadly, was in jail and their mother was lost in a world of heroin addiction and other drugs. My goal, at this time, was to keep the girls safe, within my family, the Robinson family, and not lose them to the 'system'.

I was living in Ballarat when the girls came to live with me. I cashed in my superannuation and bought us a house to keep us safe and have some security.

The next few years were fraught with pain, fear, resentment and exhaustion! However, underlying it all was the love I had for these two little girls, as well as feelings of gratitude and privilege that because of my position in life, I was able to take them into my home. I felt so thankful that I was physically and mentally able to care for them and each day became a blessing as celebrated each step we took.

The case worker who had been involved in managing the girls' case, told me it would take twelve months for the girls to accept me as their full-time carer, and as the time passed, this happened. My older granddaughter had experienced four carers in her two years of life which made me the fifth person to be looking after her.

The first lesson for me was all about providing a safe and secure environment for two little girls whose lives had been spent amid alcohol, drugs and violence and it was important to provide a safe place so that we all had somewhere to release our emotions and not worry anyone else.

Their stories contain deep pain and anguish, learning to live in a strange world with their nan, not their parents and brothers, telling of sad treatment by others, how we dealt with every day, and ways in which I attempted to help them learn to deal with this pain and deal with this absolute despair and sorrow. And above all, for me to keep them safe.

Almost immediately I learned these two little girls required a different parenting approach compared to raising my sons. They were girls and would obviously develop differently. They were my granddaughters, not my daughters, and their first loyalty would always be to their parents, no matter what happened. They were also emotionally damaged and they were living in my home with just me to look after them!

With this new responsibility, I realised I needed additional emotional support and training, so I continued to study with Nicholas de Castella, completing his breathwork therapist course. Following that, I spent other weekends at the college, helping Nicholas out on his other courses.

DAKOTA AND SUMMER

Let me paint the picture for you. Here I was, a fifty-six year-old retired school teacher, raising two little girls, both still in nappies and taking bottles. I found out very quickly who my true friends were at the time. Many didn't really want little people visiting their homes so my life became very lonely during this period. In those days, there were no support groups for people in my situation, so I helped to set up a kinship carers' support group, the first one in Ballarat. I invited other carers to join and the group grew to ten. I also continued to work as a tutor for adults and intellectually disabled people and taught tai chi every week.

It took a while for me to get to know the girls and begin to see the advantages of the emotional intelligence work I was doing with them. However, as I persevered and let go of more and more of my own expectations, our life together changed and the girls began to flower. Dakota's 'flowering' was much easier to instigate as she was an effervescent child – very open to learning and trying new things. I found she loved a challenge and responded to the emotional intelligence work early and with great gusto. She also loved to have a yell and a loud cry and I'm sure she felt the benefits of this emotional release. I felt honoured being with this child, as she allowed herself to become her own true self. I also learnt that **trust** is one of the important aspects of this work, because without trust little will happen. Equally important, was the trust Dakota had in herself so she could let her emotions go when she needed to.

The importance of trust was reinforced a few months later when the girls returned from a visit with their mother. They got out of bed and started fighting, with Dakota teasing her little sister. I yelled at her and said that she could take this behaviour to school and let her teacher deal with it, as I could not. She came over to me and burst into tears, and through her sobs explained to me, "I can't cry at Mum's, I can't cry at Dad's, or at school. This is the only place I am allowed to cry." Wow! Out of the mouth of babes! So, I put my arms around her, told her that there was an angel over my shoulder, with a bucket and she would take the tears and anger away and let it happen. She allowed herself to cry bitterly but, after it was done, she became her happy little self again.

This was one of the most important lessons for me and I have never betrayed that trust. Sometimes, when I use the girls as examples in my work with others, I always ask their permission first. When I began writing this book, I asked their permission as they have now become teenagers. Summer's only condition was that she could read the book first.

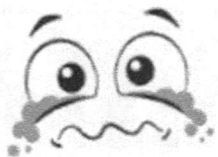

Dakota's emotional releases and growth grew dramatically from there on. She still had quiet times, where she chose to hang onto her pain, times when she slipped back into her "poor me, I don't have a family," what I refer to as, 'victim mode'. This was partly because Dakota had experienced living with her parents and older half- brothers for over a year, so this was an important issue for her and she always kept photos of her half-brothers and her father in her bedroom. Occasionally, she would cry and say how much she missed them. One day, I took a photo of the boys and asked her what this 'family' was in her life. I asked her, "Is this a real family? Do you know these people and what have you shared with them?" She faced these questions bravely, talked about her sibling and the family life she has experienced with me, and I think these discussions helped her to understand and resolve some of this pain.

In the safety of her bedroom, Dakota would let out her pain, belting the bed with her junior foam baseball bat, often using language I was not aware she even knew! However, because it was **her** room, she knew it was a safe environment and Nan supported her. She told someone once, "It's my room and I can say what I like in here. Nan said so."

During this period, we moved to another house and the girls attended a small rural school, near the mountains in Victoria's north west. As there were only a few students at the school, for

Dakota, it was a huge challenge. She became very open about her feelings, sometimes to her disadvantage. Even today, some people still believe children should be seen and not heard. Compared to the other children, Dakota was a very different soul, with an open mind to the world. Because of her background, she also had a different sense of herself, which meant she found few friends at school and became the odd one out. It was a trying few years for us all. I offered to send her to another school, but she said she felt safe at this school. Against my better judgement, I allowed her to stay for primary school and provided a safe environment for her at home, where she could vent her feelings.

I filled the girls' primary school years with study and completed a Diploma of Counselling, with the Australian Institute of Professional Counsellors. This not only gave me qualifications to be able to work as a counsellor, it also helped me understand the girls and myself a little better. I found the unit on domestic violence very confronting and I had to deal with my own feelings, resulting in seeing a counsellor myself. Living with the girls had also triggered my own feelings of abandonment, so this was another area I needed to work on. My own emotional learning and development was deepening every day.

I continued to work with my own feelings and in 2007, I discovered the 'Get Real workshops' – an Australian-wide organisation that works with young people and their carers, offering training programs around developing emotional resilience and empowerment. I also completed another course called 'The Journey' and so began another phase in my life. There were also kids' programs available and both Dakota and Summer attended several. These programs gave the girls a deeper understanding of their own actions and emotions and they're able to access this knowledge when needed.

SUMMER

Compared to Dakota, Summer has been a very different girl to work with. She was taken from her mother around six weeks of age, before the maternal bond was formed, and then put into foster care for six months, before she was returned to me, so she dealt with the world very differently. She became Dakota's shadow and it seemed like she could not live without her, until she entered her teens when she demonstrated to us that she can move on her own. Despite fighting with each other from time to time, like all siblings, the girls have a very deep bond and over the years have supported each other in many areas.

For Summer, the world was a very scary place, with her big sister representing her only security. She learned through 'imitation or observational learning' and as she developed, she copied the things her sister did. However, she did not copy the 'bad' stuff', just the 'good' and this was her way of growing. For example, Summer worked out for herself that if she had good manners, was quiet and polite, then the world would be safe. As she grew, her manners became impeccable and she developed the knack of being able to change loyalty easily, from one career to another. For example, she would visit her great-aunt and when I picked her up from there, she would not speak to me or even acknowledge I was there until we returned home. For a few days her behaviour would be terrible and she would treat me with disdain and contempt. At home, she would throw the most incredible tantrums but was always well behaved and beautifully mannered outside.

For the first two years with Summer, I felt she was hiding behind a façade. When anything went wrong and I thought she was being insolent, she showed little emotion and just looked sullen and cold.

Yes, I felt very hurt and, for her, I felt angry that the girls' parents had such power to hurt these children in this way. However, one day I followed my own intuition and discovered just what she was hiding and what she had accomplished to achieve this control over her emotions.

I listened to my heart and offered her a hug. What followed really blew me away and as this little girl screamed and cried and it was then I realised just how deep her fear was – fear of being hurt, fear of abandonment, fear of the world – and how cleverly she had hidden it from everyone around her.

Summer had also become very watchful and aware in her little world. When her sister did things that brought her praise and rewards, Summer added her own brand of 'goodness' so she received the praise and care she so longed for.

I asked her quietly if she was frightened of going to her mother. This little child just sobbed, and I knew I had broken through. She began to talk about how she was feeling, and like her big sister, she became very fond of using the foam baseball bat, swearing and yelling loudly. She would come to me and ask, "Can I use the bat? Can I leave the door open/shut?, Can I swear?"

I would listen to her screams and yells and not allow myself to become involved as this was her pain, not mine. When she had finished, she would come out for a hug and simply say, "I feel better now" and go off to whatever her next activity was. Sadly, Summer's view of herself was so flawed and it has taken a lot of time and work with me, as well as with a psychiatrist, to be able to see that the real Summer is loveable and worthwhile.

During this period, we also worked, for a long time, with a set of stacking Matryoshka dolls, also known as babushka dolls. While we played with these dolls, we would talk about how a person has so many different parts which make up the 'whole', how each part is an integral part of the person and how different each part is — not good or bad — just part of the whole person. As we took the dolls apart, I would encourage the girls to name each part. Often Summer would cry as she described her parts as nasty, spiteful or mean, so I was always sure to add loveable, clever and loving, helping her see the completeness of it all and how this was right. If she was treating Dakota badly, I sometimes I would ask her what part of her was showing today and she was always able to admit her feelings, prepared to do something about it. Even now, as a nineteen-year-old, Summer will acknowledge what is happening for her and is able to make changes for herself.

As Summer began to open her heart and allow me to see inside, I was always aware that she was wary of the chance to make changes and always very aware of just how fragile this child's emotional state was. I have felt very humble and very watchful of the steps I took as I could not afford to ever let her down.

When she was in grade six and going through typical behaviour at that age, I found she would come home from school and just go to bed, only coming out for a meal. There was little interaction with me, and I felt concerned about what was happening. I was put in contact with a local case worker/social worker who spent some time with me and told me about a disorder known as 'Reactive Attachment Disorder'. This helped explain much of Summer's behaviour and attitudes.

She is, we have now been told, on the lower end of the spectrum, however, this does impact on her life as she often appears cold and indifferent, she does not sympathise with others and tends to stand back and look on.

Early in Year 8 she asked for some counselling sessions as teenage girls were proving hard to work out, she said she was honest with these counsellors and there were some good breakthroughs – albeit slowly. She and I can now talk about how she is feeling, what is happening for her, she has cried bitterly about her so-called failure to win a boyfriend and just a while ago she showed genuine emotion for an old friend of ours who has passed over.

As Summer matures, she has begun to see herself in a more realistic light and my hopes are rising that she will keep growing. In 2018, she saved enough to go to England for three months, then got her work visa and returned for a two-year working holiday.

More recently though, her anger has begun to emerge again, and her rage frightens her. Fortunately boxing, running and sport are good outlets for her now and she is able to manage these emotions.

NIGHTLY RITUALS

I always made sure I read to the girls at night. We would sit on the floor, on a warm blanket, in one of their rooms, one on either side of me, and read together. As they grew older, I held a little ritual before bedtime whenever I could. I would take a lit candle to one of their bedrooms and we would sit in a circle around it, holding hands. One after the other we would talk about what was happening in our lives and then we would honour each other by acknowledging something about each other that gave us joy. Compliments like, "Summer's hair looks lovely since she washed it." This ritual grew as the girls matured and it helped to make bedtime a peaceful time. Sometimes we would simply meditate together or listen to a song that we all liked. During these experiences, my goal was for us to connect with each other before the day ended and provide a loving embrace for the girls to go to bed with.

MY WORK CONTINUES

I know the work with these girls is not finished but we continue to take each day as it comes and are open about our feelings. I know now that the girls are also open to counselling and as the years have passed, this has given them a solid grounding for change.

For me, the greatest part of this relationship has been the love, trust and understanding we have for each other. When I am feeling down or angry, I can tell them, and they understand. They don't run away from the feelings and they still love each other. I believe they will always need support emotionally because of their painful past and disappointments that run deep. However, **I know** they have the strength and understanding to seek help when they need to.

This is all I have – my story – a journey of pain, emotional intelligence as it happened to me, loss, betrayal, great love and huge growth – a journey that led me through this life, that opened me up in a way I could never have imagined.

As you read through this, there may be something you can use in your own life, as well as in your role as carer to your child.

There will be more on emotions later in this work and as I start, I want you to know there is **no blame** attached to anyone or anything in this story. This was my journey, to walk with the support of family and friends.

For most of my life I have strived to be true to myself, with the result it has often been a solitary path I walked because **I chose** to.

This tells of how we did this, some of the practices I used and explored, leading to skills they now have which will stand them in good stead all of their lives. It also describes how I felt during these first few years, the deep-seated emotions I needed to deal with every day and every night for so many years, and how I learned to understand what I needed to do and how to do it: to provide a safe and secure environment for two emotionally scarred children and guide them towards a happy life.

> "A person's a person, no matter how small."
>
> — DR. SEUSS

CHAPTER 2
Helping Your Child Develop Emotional Intelligence

A s you read the following chapter, I ask you to consider these questions:

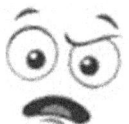

What is emotional intelligence?

What does it mean for a child?

What does it mean for me – as a parent, grandparent, for anyone caring for children?

What does it mean when I suggest you help this child, you love so dearly, to become emotionally intelligent?

What do I want for this child?

How can I provide the understanding and support this child needs to become emotionally well, and know this is okay?

How do I live my truth daily?

How do I help my children find their truth and learn to live within this truth?

*How do we all learn to **be real?***

For all my life I have felt the restrictions of other people's expectations of me. I grew up with a younger and an older sister who are the very opposite to me in many ways and was always asked, "Why can't you be more like your sisters?" I was the explorer, the one who played sport, the one who did not want to conform, who always wanted to know what was around the next corner.

Many years later, as a mother, I was also not willing to conform. "Mum, could you please wear a skirt to the parent teacher interviews?," my youngest son used to ask me when this event came around each year. I didn't own any skirts, or dresses so I couldn't do this. As we walked to school one day, and I was walking in the gutter, he told me that, "I was an embarrassment to be with", and I was, because I was different.

"Why do you need to ask so many questions?" This happened when I was working in a brake factory. I ended up lasting only two weeks in this job because I questioned the reason why I was doing what was asked of me. When I told them at the factory I wouldn't be coming back after Easter, they were shocked!

Probably, on all those occasions, I could have done what I was asked and changed my ways. I could have conformed, and, in many cases, it might have been easier for others, but not for me, as my rebellious spirit could not be crushed.

A TSUNAMI OF EMOTIONS

I began writing this book back in 2004, just after the Boxing Day Tsunami, and after witnessing four young children watch the devastation on television. I tried to answer their questions openly and honestly, whilst also being aware of the fear this disaster generated in them, and how important it was for them to be told the truth.

In fact, I was feeling very excited that I had finally begun to put down my ideas, after carrying around the hope that I could write something to help children and all who cared for them. I wanted people to learn about what emotions are and how they impact our lives.

For many years I procrastinated and went no further with this work. However, I realised there was a great need for this information and that this would be a book with a very important message. Children need to learn about emotions and know they have the ability to understand and acknowledge them. They also need to learn skills to deal with emotions in a safe and supportive environment, learning to sit with and within their feelings – giving them credence and then letting them go.

As I have worked as a therapist, completed the 'Journey Teachings' program and shared my life with two teenage girls, I have become very much aware of the children learning to cope with today's world; a world of working parents and driven by technology. I realised the skills I have learnt and developed, as well as the ideas I have about raising emotionally intelligent and resilient children, could be useful to the people whose responsibility is to care for and raise them.

Before I begin, I would like to briefly outline my beliefs on what feelings and emotions are.

Emotions are energy — energy that we store in our bodies and, if not let go, will cause pain and illness.

I use five categories for emotions.

Joy   Anger   Fear   Sadness   Nothing

Because I chose not to be like everybody else, I have led an interesting and challenging life and there is very little I would change, even if I could.

Growing up in a traditional Presbyterian household, I learned the values of home and family. I was given security, knowing that Mum and Dad would always be there for me. However, I was also the rebel, the square peg in the round hole. I fought my mother all the way to be my true self, thus developing my own inner strength at an early age.

As an adult, I also learned about the 'Enneagram' and understand that I took on an '8 personality type: The Challenger' to be able to survive. The Enneagram is a system of personality which describes people in terms of nine parts, each with their own motivations, fears and internal dynamics. Each of the nine personality types has its own driving force, which is centred around a particular emotion. Eights are self-confident, strong and assertive. They are also protective, resourceful, straight-talking, and decisive.

Even though these wonderful parents and family were my first teachers, I found myself not being accepted for who I thought I was. I wanted to be me but found myself having to fit into Mum's idea of a girl or my dad's idea of a girl. I was a tomboy, loud and intelligent, full of my own importance I suppose, and so it was impossible for me to fit into the round shape they created for me because I was 'odd- shaped'.

So, the process began of learning not to fully feel my emotions.

Anger

My dad used his belt on me three times in my life, each time when I was feeling angry and expressed it by throwing things. I learnt that anger is bad.

Sadness

I was not encouraged to cry, as "only babies cry," which meant I could not cry and allow my brother to see my pain when he teased me for being 'fat'. I learnt not to show hurt and sadness.

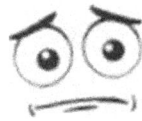

Fear and grief

When someone died, we were not involved nor was death talked about, so I was well into my twenties before I even knew what a funeral was and what happened at one. I learnt that grief is something you avoid and hide.

Joy

I was put down for being too boisterous and too happy because it was just 'not the done thing'. I learnt to not show my true personality.

There have certainly been times in my life when I have pushed down my feelings, such the resentment I felt when I became a single mother, which later escalated into deep anger.

During my time living and working in China, I purposely repressed my feelings because it was neither the time nor the place to be emotional.

As a child, school was a place I loved, because it not only challenged my mind, it also challenged me physically. I enjoyed sport immensely and was part of school teams in netball, softball and other sports. That was until I behaved 'badly' at an interschool competition when I stood up to a teacher and told her my feelings about her umpiring. My sports teacher used the most effective punishment possible and banned me from all sports for a year. She then made me sit and watch all of the games my team played.

The one positive result from this experience was that I never showed anger on a sporting field again, until I was in my late forties and realised I didn't want to do this anymore and so retired.

I do know the large amount of weekly sport I played, which kept me physically busy, also allowed me to deal with my emotions, albeit subconsciously, and so kept me out of trouble. Also, each Saturday night, after a day's sport, I would go dancing and this is one of the best ways to release energy.

I chose primary school teaching as my life's work and it fulfilled me in many ways. It was physically and intellectually challenging and I thrived in this environment. I was certainly not the best teacher around, but because I genuinely loved and trusted children, as an educator I was caring, compassionate and real. I encouraged the children's growth and sense of adventure. I also valued kindness and honesty and there was mutual respect between me and the children in my care.

Children and their development became my passion, a passion that grew throughout my life and remains just as strong today.

I had three beautiful sons who went through the usual experiences of childhood and challenges of growing up. Somehow, I realised that to deal with anger one had to be physical, so I encouraged them to throw rocks at the back fence until they felt better. As I shared my life with them, I realised just how hard it is for some children to feel safe expressing themselves. For others, the challenge is to understand their inner pain is what is holding them back – that their inner picture or themselves, their core belief, is that they are unlovable and not worth caring about.

When my youngest son went to school, I re-entered the workforce as a teacher/librarian, and later as a classroom teacher. As a divorced mother of three primary school aged children, and the family's sole provider, I felt the beginnings of a very deep sense of anger. This feeling later turned into rage because I was hanging on to and hiding the pain I felt at that stage in my life. Because I did not know any other way, I was unable to let my real feelings out.

A CHANGING WORLD

The longer I stayed in teaching, the more changes I witnessed. At the time, there was no guidance on preparing lesson plans or reading programs. There were also no spelling lists or multiplication tables.

Above all, I noticed a huge change in the school children. Gone were the days of children wanting to learn for themselves and being eager to help. Instead, I saw children with very low self-esteem, who relied on external stimuli for their entertainment, such as televisions and other electronic devices, which took the place of a child's natural desire to learn and think for themselves. With so many screens now readily available, children could now just sit back and be entertained, without putting effort into their learning.

I know a gorgeous eight-year-old who was given an iPad for Christmas, not because he needed it for school, just for fun. I also know from my work that some schools expect parents to provide computers to children as soon as they start school. This trend does worry me as many children no longer go outside to play, spending the bulk of their lives watching screens, absorbed in an alternate, artificial world.

Seeing children exposed to all this technology also brought about a change in me as an educator. I was no longer the strong, independent teacher who expected children to behave and do what they were told. I realised times had changed and that instead of expecting the children to continue learning in traditional ways, I needed to explore other approaches to learning and became a 'facilitator of learning' – sourcing the work for the children and encouraging them to choose and learn in areas they were interested in.

I have always regarded children as the greatest gift the universe has bestowed on us and I feel very humble and blessed to have raised three healthy sons myself, who have given me a deeper understanding of a child's emotional needs. I also feel very privileged to have had the experience of being a teacher of small children, sharing their lives and their growth.

The world has certainly changed for our children and it has become much harder to provide outdoor activities for some. When I visited a friend last year her twenty-two-year old son spent the whole time I was there on the computer, chatting with his 'friends' and not conversing at all with us. My own granddaughters spend much of their time on their phones, in their rooms and not going out.

As such, I applaud the parents who find activities for their children so they can be active. It is never easy to be a parent and, as I age and observe, I feel the world is getting harder for those who just want the best for their children.

> "There can be no keener revelation of a society's soul than the way in which it treats its children."
>
> — NELSON MANDELA, FORMER PRESIDENT OF SOUTH AFRICA

CHAPTER 3
In My Classroom

As a primary school teacher, it was my experience that my colleagues were usually considerate of a child's feelings, but only to a point. With large classes to manage every day, it's often easier for teachers to keep children on the same, safe emotional level. This means keeping their classroom calm and neutral. This occurs sometimes when a teacher has had no real experience dealing with their own, or other people's emotions.

The challenge for teachers is that we have no idea what has happened to the child before they arrive at school each day. Unless something is reported to us, we just take it for granted that the child is happy. Something may have also happened in our own lives, before we came into the classroom, something that makes us less open to the children we were responsible for.

I had one experience in my second year out of teachers' college that I've never forgotten. I was teaching in a small school, with only two teachers and thirty students – from prep to year two. One morning, a little girl in prep arrived at school and announced, "My Daddy belted Mummy last night, he took all of our money and now he is gone." From this experience, I learned to look carefully at children before we started teaching day and tune in to those I thought were in need of extra support.

I also know from my own experience, when there had been an upset in my home that I was feeling anxious about, I needed to feel confident I was emotionally stable enough to be with the children.

However, as within the home environment, it is possible to work with children in the classroom to help them understand their feelings as well as begin to develop and further their emotional intelligence.

As a grandparent, I rejoice when I see the introduction of wellness programs such as – 'Seasons for Growth', 'Cool Kids', 'Wellness Places', 'The Journey' and similar, introduced into our Victorian schools. Elsewhere, in Queensland, there are the 'Get Real' and 'Real Kids,' helping kids. This is a very exciting development for our children as it's providing them with safe places to grow and emotionally develop.

Many schools now place a value on education around emotional intelligence, even though some of it comes under different names. I know beautiful people who run regular workshops for children and teenagers so they also have access to places of learning for emotional wellness. Many schools also have wellness centres within the school buildings. My hope is that the people who run these centres are aware of how vulnerable children and teens are and are able to provide the support they need.

My own experience has been that some teachers can be reluctant to begin any work that involves exploring children's emotions. I remember suggesting to the principal of one of the small schools I taught at, that we provide a punching bag and regular supervised opportunities to use it for a student whose parents had recently separated. He thought it was a good idea and "would probably help", but "it was too radical for our school".

COLOURS, MUSIC AND JOY BREAKS

When I first began to widen my own personal growth experiences, I was in a small, rural school and was responsible for teaching eighteen children in a multi-age group, from years three to six. There was one other teacher and an aide. Over two years, nine of these children experienced a death within their family group, including the loss of a father, a baby sister and grandparents. I observed these children in their grief and the impact it had on the rest of the class and knew I needed to provide a place where the children could safely acknowledge and experience their emotions.

In the past, I had attended 'Passionately Alive' workshops with Nicholas de Castella and I knew the techniques I had learnt could be adapted to the classroom.

Firstly, I moved the children's individual desks into a circle so that each child could see everyone else. I introduced the program to the children, explained the process and the desired goal of the program. I explained to the children that they would not be asked to do anything they felt was not okay, and that it was an opportunity for some personal growth. I then asked the children for input and told each of them to let their parents know what was happening. In hindsight, it would have been a better idea to have had a parent information night where I could explain what I had told the children.

Together, the children and I worked out some guidelines and discussed important issues, such as confidentiality, trust, truth and honouring each other. Because I had already taught these children for two years, the trust had been established.

I had also worked with a program called, 'Feelings and Colour' in my classroom for many years so the children were familiar with it. This program is based on the many aspects of the four groups of feelings we experience, which are linked with colour, art and music and had many colourful interpretations of this work decorating the walls of our classroom.

Each morning, after the physical start to the day, the children and I would sit in a circle on the carpeted floor so that each person could see each other's face. At the beginning, I would ask the children to close their eyes and become aware of where they were. When we close our eyes, we shut out the world around us and this helps to bring our awareness to within ourselves. It also stops us getting distracted. I would then ask the children to become aware of the rhythm of their breathing and to deepen it, if they could. I then asked them how they were feeling at that moment.

With open eyes, the children were then each encouraged to share how they were feeling, in a single word if they were able. If not, I would encourage them to just try and explain how they were feeling and then, perhaps a word would come. So, we would go around the circle and each person, including me, had an opportunity to express their feelings. At the end of each person's sharing, I would quietly thank the child, whilst keeping eye contact. Some of the boys took a little longer to explain their feelings but I let them know that it was okay for them to say they didn't know. The words did come, eventually, and it was exciting to be a part of this sharing time. At the end of the sharing, the children could ask questions before they chose the next step, which had to involve music. Mostly this was 'mad' dancing!

After the first few days of shyness and lots of giggling, the children began to look deeper within themselves and were able to express exactly how they felt. One day a little girl in my class said, "I feel angry and I want to dance to loud music"... and so we did.

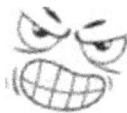

At the beginning of the program, I let the children use eye masks to help them feel anonymous and less inhibited. However, this only lasted a few days before the children chose to discard them.

The dance part for me was very important as we could physically release any energy we had. The dancing ranged from slow graceful moves, to loud staccato type jumps and other actions. This was also a time without talking and the children loved this part – they became freer and more energetic, with this experience moving them so much.

At the end of the music, the children would put their desks back in place, begin work and the day would flow from there. If a problem arose, we would deal with it together and the children became most adept at making decisions and imposing consequences.

During the day we would also have regular 'joy breaks'. The children would stop work, stand up, ready to move, while a chosen volunteer would provide the activity for the class. It may be something like dancing, smiling at each other, or walking around the room sideways, any way to get the children moving and give their brains a break. The time limit was five minutes and then they would return to their work. It was good stuff!

CHILDREN AND GRIEF

Late in the second year a beloved grandmother died after an unexpected short illness and her two grandchildren were devastated. It was so gratifying for me to be a part of a supportive and compassionate group who walked beside these children at this difficult time. Their mother brought up a book designed for children to work through grief and this was included as part of our daily schoolwork.

I did ruffle feathers with this work and, in hindsight, I should have gone to the school council and explained what I wanted to do, the process involved and asked for their support. But I didn't because I knew how good it was and perhaps I just wanted to be left alone to experiment with it. My colleagues did not approve of what I was doing and only two parents objected. Interestingly, these same parents were in a difficult marriage, so I knew this was confronting for them, however, as they didn't come and talk to me about it, I couldn't follow this up with them. As a result, their children sat out on the sidelines and watched, as they weren't allowed to participate. Perhaps they absorbed something from the sidelines. Many years later, the marriage broke up — anger, alcohol and sadness were the cause. Maybe these parents could have been helped through some of the work I was doing with the children?

At the time, I felt so passionate about helping these children understand the grieving process, also their own feelings relating to that, and I know how wonderful this program was for them.

Since leaving the classroom, I am even more passionate about this work but I also realise that teachers, like parents, need to confront their own feelings, their own fears, so the work can be mutually worthwhile.

OUR BEAUTIFUL TEENS

Over the years, as I reared the next generation, I have learned that many of these lessons and teachings continue to be crucial, as kids grow into teenagers, and then into adults.

It's so important to tell a teenager how wonderful they are, how beautiful, how clever, and how important they are to you as a parent. Teenage years are so fraught with negatives, put downs and other pressures so it's easy for a young person to lose sight of how special they really are.

Teenagers are really just big kids – kids who are growing through a transition period in their lives, where self-beliefs are constantly challenged and so much pressure is put on them to be just like everybody else. This, in itself, is a fallacy because each teenager is unique, special and loveable just as they are – not as we want them to be, but just as they are.

As parents, it is a privilege to walk beside these beautiful people, to share their dreams, their losses and their triumphs and to just **be there.** Teenagers need us, to talk with us and have us **hear** them, to accept them as they are and not to judge.

We need to remember that we were all where they are now and have survived – with help and support, they too will grow through these years if we can but let go of the need to control and just accept our kids for who they are.

It is sometimes difficult for us as parents not to judge what is happening with our teenagers, difficult to let go of the control we would like over them, but we must. We must give them our love and support to survive these years.

My granddaughters and I have survived these years and I are deeply grateful for the work we have done together and the respect the girls have shown for this work – I rejoice when I see them using techniques I have taught them in their everyday lives.

They still need my support as their early emotional lives were so impacted, but they can see this emotional need in others and they also can see the need for support within themselves. It's fascinating to hear about the challenges their friends are having in their lives and how they have counselled them. Dakota has a friend who invites violent men into her life and although it rings loud alarm bells for my grand-daughter, her friend doesn't understand what she's doing. I just smile as Dakota talks – she has it and I'm grateful.

I have purposely not written about drugs and the part it can play in many lives, the dangers, the destructiveness, the fear, the anger and the loss – it is too deep for me here and this book is not the place. I do plan one day to write about my experiences and what they have taught me. There are so many great books about this problem and even today I am still learning.

> "Children must be taught HOW to think, not WHAT to think."
>
> — MARGARET MEAD, CULTURAL ANTHROPOLOGIST

CHAPTER 4

I'm a Carer – How Can I Help the Child in My Life?

Some of the ideas I talk about in this book may prove confronting to some as they may bring up other issues. We all have issues from our earlier life we think we have dealt with, or perhaps buried and ignored. However, this is not a bad thing because if you do carry 'baggage' from the past, your life will become easier and lighter when we let go of it.

If it becomes a problem for you, please find a counsellor, or someone you trust, to talk through these issues. I remember when the girls first came to live with me and we began dealing with their issues around abandonment, I felt an emotional trigger. This suggested to me I had touched on my own abandonment issues, so I found a counsellor and talked things through with her. It's important to find someone you can share your feelings with and explore your past emotions, as well as your understanding of these.

This work cannot succeed unless you're truly sincere in your desire to help your child and prepared to grow alongside them. We can't force children to do this work as they will resist, and you will lose the opportunity to help them. Sometimes, you can do this work without any explanation and be guided by the child.

For example, recently my grandson came to visit, and he was very angry with his mum. I put on the hand protector glove and invited him to punch it as hard as he could, which he did. He then used his feet to kick the glove. After a few minutes, when his anger was spent, he didn't need to talk about it, he just needed to release the emotion.

As the relationship and trust between you grows and if your child is old enough to understand, I advise you to talk with them and explain what you're going to do. I did this with my granddaughters when they were very young and, for us, it worked. Much of this work can be done easily and incorporated into everyday activities. It does not need to be heavy and serious. Be aware that sometimes your own fear may be aroused and this is quickly picked up by your child. Similarly, if you are not truly present and committed to this work, the task will be sabotaged.

Being present means being fully aware of the space you are in — feeling emotions as they happen, acknowledging what is happening and being in the moment. It's all about being mindful of where you are, of what's happening and not letting your mind wander away from the task at hand.

So, how and where do you start emotionally connecting with your child?

Once you have decided that you are prepared to share feelings with your child, put aside a short time during the day when you can plan what needs to be dealt with and how you are going to go about it. This can be done so incidentally, throughout the day, and with practice, it becomes second nature.

Begin by facing your own fears and the reasons they are there. Ask yourself: *What are the deepest fears I have and how can I let them go?*

Acknowledge your own feelings and accept they are part of who you are and know that you can be more real when you allow yourself to see who you really are. You may find parts of yourself that have been hidden, so welcome them in and feel how they feel.

To help you do this, find a quiet place and allow yourself a few minutes of solitude. Close your eyes and become aware of your breath, following it in and out as you breathe. Ask yourself: *What am I feeling right now?* Allow yourself to be patient and let the feelings arise. Even if there is only a tiny whisper of a feeling, let it rise. Acknowledge this feeling and give it a name. To let it go, breathe into the feeling and relax as you breathe it out through your mouth. Repeat this until you feel you have let it go.

It's important that you are honest with yourself before you can be honest with a child. Children see right through people who are not truthful, and you lose trust.

Believe in what you are doing. If this is what you want for your child, then have faith. Don't beat yourself up and find fault with yourself. Children are forgiving and they know when people really care. In fact, sometimes you can talk to your child about your fears around this and this will only deepen the experience.

Listen to yourself and to your reactions. List the things you'd like for the child to be able to achieve by acknowledging their feelings, deciding which ones you can deal with and which ones you cannot. Begin with the easier ones so you get a little practice before the bigger and more complex ones arise. Death and sex are sometimes big issues for parents, as they tend to confront our fears and our own upbringing.

Learn to say **sorry** when you are wrong, hurtful or thoughtless and mean it. Don't say it if you don't mean it. Many children never learn that parents can be wrong too and it is validating for the child to have this shared with them. Sorry is often one of the hardest words to say to anyone and it is much harder to say it to a child. Once you start, however, it becomes part of daily life and this is a sign of being real. When my son is tired or stressed, he often gets angry but later he will apologise for this and explain what's happening for him.

Accept your child as they are. Before you begin this process with your child, be completely honest with your feelings about them. Don't try to change things you don't like in them. Perhaps these things are resonating with a part of you that you do not like in yourself. You may find that as you work, these settle themselves, or you may have to find help for yourself. Unlike the past, seeking help from professionals is far more accepted and counsellors are usually warm and ready to support you.

DECIDE NOT TO JUDGE – LISTEN AND HEAR

If you need to talk about it with someone else, find a willing ear and tell the child you are doing this as well as why. It is sometimes hard when you do not like a particular friend your child has, or something has happened you're not happy about. However, it's important for you to hear the child and understand their side. Make sure you reassure the child that you are not breaking their confidence, or you will lose their trust. You do not have to like all of their friends but if they are in the child's life you need to know about each one. In fact, often friends will give you valuable insights into your child and tell you what they're really like.

As a child begins this work there may be times of stress when you do not like what the child is saying. Perhaps, you think you have the answer, but you need to learn not to judge responses as 'bad' or 'good'. This is what the child believes at that moment and they need to know you accept this.

There is no right or wrong to feelings. They are just energy and by accepting them as such we do not judge at all.

Learn to **hear** what is coming out. Sometimes a child will give you an insight into the real reason and we pass it up as it does not seem right to us.

One night Summer was very angry and belting her foam baseball bat on the bed. I asked her if she was feeling angry. "Yes!" she shouted as she bashed her bat. "Are you angry with me?" I asked. "No," she replied, bashing the baseball bat again. "Are you angry with Dad?" "No," she shouted, bashing the bat again. "Are you angry with Mum?" "Yes!" she said, as she bashed the bat on the bed again. I accepted her answer and encouraged her to continue. However, when she was finished, she said she was still feeling angry.

Later, I talked the incident over with another counsellor and she suggested that I could have gone through the questions again, as I had only worked through the top layer. Maybe it was me she was angry with? This would have been quite understandable as I am the one person she is frightened of losing.

Later on, I learned about the process of going through the layers of emotion and it's an effective way to access the deepest of feelings. Just ask the child to really feel the feeling and then to look further into it and see if there is anything underneath.

Often anger is the first response and when the child is able to go deeper there may be fear or sadness – emotions we don't deal with very well in our everyday lives.

One important thing I have learned is that when a child has a real release of feelings, there is a peacefulness that shows through afterwards. You can actually see this inner quietness and the child tends to return to 'normal' very quickly. They may tell you, "I feel so much better now! There's no hardness in my body anymore."

Play games with your child about their feelings. Life is not meant to be always heavy and serious. Often we can help children to lift their spirits, as we support them to heal and deal with the challenges of everyday life. For example, see who can laugh, yell, sing the loudest.

We lived in a small bush area for a few years and the girls found life difficult at times. As I drove them to school, I would ask them what we could do to change the feelings we had. Sometimes we, myself included, yelled all the way to school, which was a nine kilometre trip! Other times, we laughed hilariously, we screamed, we told people off, anything to release the energy.

It's important to validate the child and honour them for being who they are. It doesn't take much to tell a child that they're wonderful, that they look great and fill your life with joy. I tell my little granddaughter every time she holds my hand how lucky I am and how great that feels. Can you remember how many times your parents told you that you were wonderful?

Start now with your own child!

When you start this work, I suggest you draw up your own guidelines with the children you're caring for. **Appropriateness is the key word here.**

It is not appropriate to yell and scream at school, in the supermarket, or in situations where there are people present who do not understand what you're doing, often relatives.

I have since learned that parents with autistic children can have cards to give out when a meltdown happens so people understand and are sensitive to the situation. This same method can be used with all children as it acknowledges that an emotional release is happening and you are there to make sure the child is safe and understood.

For the children in my care, I made their bedrooms a safe environment for each of them — a space for them to release their emotions and to be real. Each child is able to take themselves off to their bedroom for some yelling and whatever else they need to release the energy. I asked them to warn me before they began so I could reassure any other people in the house and let them know what was happening.

In this situation, no one would go in and tell them to stop and I did not allow myself to be drawn into the emotion that was being expressed. This was sometimes hard but a very necessary part of this process. The children know I'm there and would come if they called me.

Dakota said to someone one day, "I say some awful things in my room". "Do you?" they replied. "Yes, and Nanny says it's okay. It's my room and I can do what I like in here just as long as I don't break anything," Dakota told them. How's that for faith and trust in a child!

This experience gave Dakota the knowledge that it's okay to let go of emotions in a safe environment and that there will be no consequences. However, one time, she did break her coat hooks off the wall. Later, when we talked about it, she was able to see that she hadn't done the right thing because she now had no hooks to hang her clothes. From this experience, I taught the girls about choice and consequence and it didn't take them long to understand this concept.

There have only been a few occasions, when Dakota has been very tired or concerned about what's happening in her dad's life, that the explosions occurred elsewhere. Her schools have had to deal with a few outbursts, but because I had explained to the teachers the work I was doing with the girls, there was usually understanding and support from the staff, not punishment.

For me, this is has always been a very important aspect of being a parent. I believe it's important for a child's teacher to be kept informed about what's happening in their lives, so that support and understanding can be given when needed. I remember, as a teacher, children coming to school in the morning like thunder, as if they had the weight of the world on their shoulders, and I would wonder what they had experienced before coming to school.

We don't know what happens at homes before children come to school yet we expect them to be well behaved and ready to learn, when perhaps what they actually need is understanding and the time and space to let it all go. A hug would have been the answer once, but unfortunately this is now illegal.

CHOICE AND GRATITUDE

Allowing your child choice is important. When possible, let your child pick out their own clothes when shopping. Admittedly, buying clothes can be a nightmare, especially when the parent **demands** the child buys what the parent wants them to wear. When I went shopping with the girls I found it so much easier and, in fact, very interesting, to allow them to select their own clothes. This gives the child the opportunity to develop their own sense of style and colour and it also helps them to understand that being told 'no' is okay.

Thank the child for what they do and give to you. For example, one of my grandchildren complimented me when they said, "Nan, you look great for your age." "Thanks," I replied gratefully. Also thank children for the chores they do so they know what they do is worthwhile. The other day I thanked my three-year-old grandson for coming with me to the pool, "because I had so much fun," I told him. He looked at me a little puzzled and said "Why are you thanking me?" Why shouldn't we thank our children?

Introduce the child to her breathing. Our breath is our lifeline to mental, emotional and physical balance so if we can help children become aware of their breath at an early age, they will also learn about the power of the breath.

For example, slowing down the breath can bring relaxation. Breathing in deeply and exhaling quickly can release energy. Holding the breath can help to clear the mind.

Practise by:

- **Pretending to blow out candles in short sharp, staccato bursts.**
- **Blowing a feather from your hand to the ceiling, alternating with light puffs, long puffs and strong breaths.**

- **Blow up a balloon and use your hands to show how big it can get.**
- **Puff out in short puffs on a dandelion.**

These can all be done seriously or as a fun activity.

As children grow, it is also helpful to let them explore the spiritual side of their lives because this also plays a very important part in our overall development. For me, this does not necessarily mean religion, just the parts of me that keep my feet on the ground. These are the beliefs I have around the world and what it holds and the inner knowledge that I can do this. This will be different for many of us and sometimes it is the deepest part of us. I believe we can help our children understand that the world we live in is only one facet of life, that spiritual beliefs are important and encourage them to develop their own.

I hope I have given you an introduction to some important concepts that will help your child to develop and become emotionally aware. I have tried all of these ideas, so I know they work and the benefit they offer.

I think the one important point here is that **you,** as a carer, feel comfortable in what you are trying to do and that you learn to relax, allowing your child to sometimes set the pace and accept what happens. Open your mind and your heart to your child, show them how you feel, warts and all. Accept how they feel and talk about it together. Communication is the key to success here.

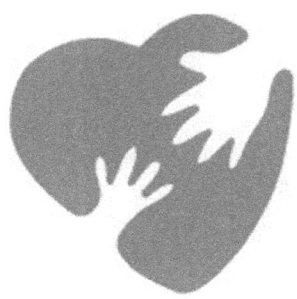

> "Who more than the defenceless and the fragile young need to be defended and protected."
>
> POPE JOHN PAUL

"Hugs can do great amounts of good, especially for children."

DIANA, PRINCESS OF WALES

CHAPTER 5
Building Trust in Children

Building trust in children is so important when it comes to teaching them how to understand and manage their emotions.

The following strategies are just some of the many ways a child can be encouraged to release their emotions, without explicitly telling them that this is the goal. You can never start too young as little children also have unspent emotions they need to release.

In the beginning, you may find yourself having to join in too. You can do these activities in the bath, in the car, outside, or in any other place that's appropriate and suitable. Public places, such as the supermarket, are not suitable environments.

Just remember, it's the child's release you're after. You can join in and lose some of your unspent energy, releasing it fully later when the time is right for you. Don't put it off though because it's important for your child that you're free and fully engaged.

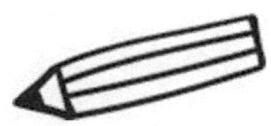

CREATING

For some of the activities it's important to set up the environment so the child feels safe and can be understood and honoured. Drawing is a great activity because you can encourage your child to talk as they draw. Use different types of medium, such as a combination of pencils, chalk and crayons. Pastels are also good as you can spread the colour out with your fingers and fists. Make no judgement about the drawing, just praise your child for doing a great job and allow them to talk about the drawing if they want to. Date each piece and keep them so you can both look back at their work when you want to. Finger paint using hands and feet is another great activity to do with children.

Make buildings with Lego and other blocks, both small and large. Buy small marbling kits for your child and decorate different size pieces of paper. Allow them to dry and make them into little books to represent feelings.

One day with her therapist D akota made a little book aboutme that just blew me away with her insights. As for her mother, she wrote that she knew "nothing more than she's happy," and mentioning her father, she wrote "I'd hate to think how he feels inside". What amazing insight for a young child!

Clay play or play dough, where figures can be made and maybe talked about is another great activity.

Use materials from around the house to make models. For example, cover a foam ball with wool, for hair, and drape material for a dress to represent a monster under the bed, or even scrunch up a piece of paper and tie it in a man's handkerchief.

Role play anything the child suggests. Sometimes it is within role play that unspoken truths appear. Be very watchful during this time and note what you see. Also, remember not to make judgements – these are the child's emotions, not yours.

Using hand puppets is a great way to take the child ' out of themselves' and to use the voice of the puppet to express what they cannot.

Sand and water play are often the most underestimated tool we all have. My grandson loves to play in water and at home his parents give him water in the sink and food colouring to make it more exciting. Give your child a variety of simple kitchen tools to play with in the water and don't mind if it spills on the floor. You can both wipe it up later. A small desk sandbox can also be useful. Put in small animals and objects and allow the child to play in it. Encourage them to tell you what they are doing. Large outside sandpits are also a fantastic place for play at any age.

Doing simple woodwork with hammers and saws, under adult supervision, is another great activity to do with children.

Use your voice to encourage them to use theirs. This is an effective way to move energy. On the way to school, I would often ask the girls, "What way would you like to do it today?" They knew I was referring to 'voice movement'. We would all laugh, sing, shout, cry as loudly as we could, all the way to school. This was great fun and I could then continue on to work knowing the girls were emotionally ready to meet the day.

You can dance and move to music in a lot of different creative ways. It may be a good idea to introduce masks in the beginning to overcome initial shyness. As the child's confidence grows, you will notice they often stop wearing the masks which encourages openness.

Don't be afraid to experiment with all different types of music – anything that will get the child moving. I would encourage the children in my classroom to, "let the music come in through your ears and out through your body". I would also encourage them to dance in different ways, to different types of music – madly and loosely, jerkily, like a robot, smoothly, any way you can make the body move. In the early days, the girls and I loved using a Celine Dion song. As it started playing, I would hear little feet pounding down the passageway as the girls rushed to join in.

Painting to music is another wonderful activity to do with children. I offered the children four different genres for their painting, or used pastels, and then chose different styles of music, depending on the emotion. The William Tell Overture is great for passion, or you can play 'dark' music, contrasted with soft gentle music, depending on the situation. If possible, let the children hear as many types of music you're able to offer.

Singing with the children, especially songs they can relate to, is another great outlet. Do all the funny actions as you sing and make the songs entertaining – little ones love to be a bit naughty and laugh loudly, particularly when they can relate to the song. One great action song that has been around for years, and still much loved by children, is the 'Hokey Pokey'. Children love to join in, and you can make it such fun!

You can also make up songs about you and them – it doesn't matter if it's not in key, just get the children involved.

USING SOUND AND MOVEMENT

It's important when someone is releasing energy to use their voice as this brings the emotion up from the base and allows it to escape. When the girls first came to live with me, instead of shouting, which would have frightened them, I used to 'sound' in the shower. This allowed me to take my awareness to the deepest part of me, giving it a sound, bringing that sound out and allowing it to escape.

Here are some effective techniques you can do with children to help them release energy through sound. Allow the children to choose which one they'd like to try:

- **Stand with your feet still and only move your body.**
- **Lie on the floor with closed eyes and allow the body to move at will.**
- **Stamp to loud music. Maybe later you can help them to find the beat and to stamp and yell.**
- **Bang a drum, tambourine, tambour, softly and then loudly.**
- **Use floaty scarves to wind around you as the music plays.**
- **Make up your own music, experimenting with your own ideas and see what happens.**
- **Shout and yell loudly. This can be introduced as a game – ask the children, "who can yell the loudest?" and don't be afraid to join in.**
- **Yell in the car, if you can stand it! This is very satisfying when you cannot see the child's face so there's a certain amount of freedom.**

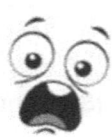

RELEASING ENERGY

Hit a ball with a bat. My dad showed me how to put a tennis ball in a stocking, hang it from the outside roof edge and use a tennis racquet. I spent many hours hitting the ball, even though I never have played tennis. Nowadays there are Totem tennis sets and tennis balls on return strings children can use.

Punch a pillow or a large cushion. This works wonders if you can get the child to verbalise or make some sound, or yell at someone they feel angry with, even if it's you. Start them off with punching the fists on the pillow saying, "I feel angry. I feel angry", and it can soon become real. I allow the children to use any language here as some words just explode when given a voice – as long as the child already knows about appropriateness.

Hit a cushion or a bed with a bat. Children's toy baseball sets can be bought for around ten dollars and, as they are light, they are perfect for this. Discuss with your child the safe use of the bat beforehand and difference between this activity and the actual violence of hitting. Find a safe place that is easily accessible for the child, away from the living part of the household, but within your hearing, and encourage them to let it all go. Keep the bats in a special place and explain to the child that they are not to be used as toys.

Put up a punching bag, buy some gloves and introduce it to your child with simple explanations about how to use it. Have a set of gloves and a receiving set, as they do in boxing gyms, and allow your child to punch and yell.

Older children can chop wood and kindling. My teenage stepdaughter used this method often to release her emotions.

Put up a target on an outside wall and encourage the child to throw the ball as hard as possible.

Encourage your child to kick a ball. I spoke earlier about the young boys I taught, from Queensland, who kicked all of our school balls over the fence, during recess.

Join in with your child when it is appropriate. This will allow you to let down the adult 'walls' and the need to control. It also gives your child permission to let go and they love to see adults being 'silly'.

Find a stick and hit a fence post. Throw rocks at the back fence, or throw balls at walls, or cricket stumps. Throwing stones seems to be a natural habit for boys and I smile every time I observe little boys doing this.

A friend of mine once went to an op shop and bought a box of old crockery and had great pleasure smashing it all on the ground. The clearing up afterwards was also 'therapeutic'.

GUARDIAN ANGELS

Older children can be encouraged to write in a personal journal and know their privacy will be respected.

Smaller children can have a journal too and they can draw pictures or just scribble. Make sure you date each piece for future reference.

If your teenager is having friendship issues, encourage them to bring the person they're having a problem with into their minds and then express exactly what it is they want to say to them. Get them to say it out loud and say everything that needs to be said. If you're working with them and they slow down, ask them, "what else needs to be said?" If they are working alone, they can be told this beforehand.

Use angels or some other magical character, such as Spiderman, to help children feel safe releasing their emotions. I told Dakota once that when she needed a cry, the angels were waiting over my shoulder with a big bag they would hold the pain in and then take it away to dispose of. She would cry so loudly and, many times, the depth of her anguish was awesome. However, when she was finished, she would stay quietly leaning on me, within my enfolding arms, until she was ready to move. Another time, when she yearned for her separated older brothers, I suggested she ask the angels to go to the boys and take them her love, which also brought her some peace.

Find a guardian angel for your child. My great grandmother held a special place in my heart as she was a true pioneer. She landed in Australia, at Portland, and then walked overland to the goldfields at Ararat. When Dakota was studying this part of Australian history at school, I was able to bring my great grandmother into her life as her guardian angel. One of my beautiful cousins sent us a photo which became a very special part of Dakota's life – her guardian angel was there to confide in and provide support. Introducing any outside support can aid release – it could be angels, a child's secret friend, a transformed friend, or something within the child's frame of reference. Let's face it, we sometimes need all the help we can get.

When there is a specific person involved, such as a guardian angel or a secret friend, put two chairs facing each other, sit the child in one and ask them to mentally 'invite' the other person to sit down so the spirit of the person is there. This removes fear from the exercise as your child can 'see' the person but there is no danger from the actual person. Encourage your child to tell the person exactly what has happened, how they're feeling, what they would like the person to know and how to help them.

THE SEVEN CIRCLES OF TRUST

Use the 'seven circles of trust' to allow your child to explore who they do and don't trust. This is a great way for some children to see their life and the people in it. Draw seven circles within each other, starting with small and growing large. Together, with the child, write down all the people in your child's life they think of then talk about how they trust these people. Allow the child to then place each person in a circle, depending on the amount of trust they have with each one. The inner circle is for the most trusted people in their lives, and the trust lessens with each widening circle, with the outer circle holding the people the child trusts the least. Be aware that each time you do this the circles may change. In my work with young children I actually only use three circles – the most trusted, ones they are not totally sure of and those they do not trust at all. This can be added to as the child matures.

Buy a set of Russian nesting dolls. I have found these to be one of my best aids and I have used them many times, with a variety of children. This activity can help your child to understand that they are not two dimensional and that we all have many facets to our characters – we need the 'good' and the 'bad' to make us balanced and a whole person. I explain that this whole doll is me and as I take off each layer I give each layer a name – for example, this is my crazy part, this is my nasty part, this is my loving part, and so on, until I reach the tiny doll at the centre which I call my soul, or the very essence of me. As I put the doll back together, we talk about each one and the part it plays in our lives. I then invite the child to do the same and name their own parts.

It's important to keep an open mind and a look out for other ideas you may be able to use with your child. If one works and it is good for you both then use it often. As my granddaughters have grown into teenagers, I continue to be very much part of their lives and am still able to use skills we have shared before. For example, recently, on the way to her karate class, I asked Dakota to close her eyes, tune in and tell me what her deepest fear was today and she did this easily. Once it is acknowledged and allowed to have its voice, an emotion can pass and be let go.

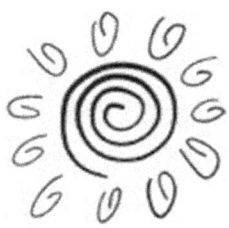

CHAPTER 6
Finding Your Centre

What do I mean by the word 'centre'?

What do you think I mean?

As a child growing up, I was a member of a Presbyterian church which I attended every Sunday, until I left home. For many years after that I regularly attended church and sent my sons to Sunday school every week. Eventually, I became very disillusioned by seeing members of the church who made rules that suited the group. These were not God's rules, and I didn't understand, nor agree with them. As a result, I left the church altogether and have not returned.

For all those years, I believed I had a soul and I don't suppose I ever questioned what that really meant. It seemed to be my base support and I became who I was because of my religious upbringing. However, after many years of broken marriages and lost hopes, I realised one day there was something in me that kept me together, kept me going when everything around me was falling away. So, I began to seek answers for other aspects of my life, such as the way I dealt with loss, the way I could always keep smiling, or, as I read once, how "I could survive a night of loneliness and pain".

It was an interesting journey to find out what it was that kept me together and, as always, things happen as they're needed. Recently, at tai chi, the ladies and I were talking about what holds us together after life events tear us apart. We all agreed there is a part of the human psyche that's indestructible.

So why not teach this to children — teach them to understand they are capable of withstanding the world and its hurts and that if they can learn to relax and find their own 'centre', whatever choices they make, they can 'ride the waves'.

I learnt and taught tai chi for many years and, my local community, recently introduced a new class for seniors. I also discovered karate in my late fifties, allowing me to embrace more Eastern philosophies. I truly felt these experiences widened my mind and opened up possibilities I had never considered before. I love some of the Eastern beliefs and have become so much more accepting of life and able to let go of unnecessary things.

When my son was deeply into drugs, I felt myself being drawn along with him. I had rented a house so he would have a home and we lived together. I realised that I was becoming codependent and actually enabling him and his habit — allowing him to walk in and out as he wanted, use my car, use drugs at home, accepting that he was a drug addict. One day, as I watched him injecting himself, I realised that, if this was what I was allowing, I was becoming an addict myself and I knew I had to get out of this precarious situation.

I moved out of the house and visited a counsellor friend of mine who explained how necessary it was for me to stay within my centre emotionally, and to not get drawn into the chaos of others' lives and problems. She taught me the importance of being able to stay within myself and deal with life's challenges, calmly and carefully. It takes a good deal of practise to find this space, but it is achievable.

As I began to study this aspect, I realised what a huge amount of garbage I had to let go of. I had spent so many sleepless nights worrying about things I could not control, that were not really any of my business. I realised I was unable to control anybody else's business and problems but my own.

So, for me, this became a journey into myself, until I found my centre – the very place where I resided and could find sustenance and power in my everyday life. I found that I could deal with the ups and downs of life better from this point. I could stay safe emotionally and I was not being drawn into other people's games and problems.

I also realised that if I could introduce children into their points of centre, then they too could develop an awareness of who they really are and that they did not have to be on emotional edge all of the time.

I am not suggesting you share this concept with your four-year-old as they are probably too young to fully understand it. However, you can teach little children simple breathing techniques to help them to relax and reach their centre. Encourage them to breathe deeply down to the point, near the tummy button, and let it go slowly. What I have learnt through practicing tai chi, is that this point is called the *tan tien* and it's the centre of gravity in the body supposedly where the chi is stored, chi being the inner energy we all have. Encourage your child to put their hand on this point, about three centimetres below the tummy button, breathe in deeply and see if they can push the hand out with their breath, then breathe out as slowly as they can.

I believe my centre is truly the deepest part of me, of my soul - the place within me that is my very core and the part that holds my faith and knowledge – knowledge that I do not walk in this world alone, that I do have a very special purpose for being here. When

I trust in this knowledge and believe that the world is a great place, then all falls into place.

INTRODUCING THE CONCEPT OF CENTRE TO A CHILD?

For the children, I introduce the idea of a very magical place inside each one of us where everything is beautiful and perfect. This is the place where all of your beautiful and fantastic ideas come from and where you can go when you are feeling unsafe, sad or fearful. In this magical place, you can find the power and strength to keep going, even though your world seems to be falling apart. I use the little Russian stacking dolls, with their tiny centre, to illustrate this.

As children mature, this can be refined and presented at whatever level the child is able to understand. Some children need to see their power as being used for their own good. For instance, when a child has been put down by others and is feeling lesser, we can talk to them about that special place inside where they have this supply of power and where the child knows they are perfect just as they are. *The Karate Kid* movies are a great example of this. This centre is the place where anyone can go when they need to feel strong and safe and you can talk with them about this – "Feel the energy you have, know you are strong and powerful, trust in your very own self as you are perfect just as you are."

Our little boys do not need to feel they need to be overpowering and bullies, nor do they need to feel they can be bullied. They just need to have trust in themselves.

Older children can be asked to describe their centres if they feel like it – "Where is it? What does it look like? What do you feel when you go in there?"

However, do not ask these questions if the child does not want to tell you. In these situations, maybe they could draw it for you. Explain to the child – "It's not your heart, it is a very special place where you can access your own power, any time you want."

Once, when I was teaching tai chi in a rural setting, I was verbally abused by a woman who asked me how I dared to say the practice had no religious connotations and suggested we had our own inner power. She argued, "there was only God's power in this world," and I acknowledged this as her true belief. However, I also see that, if I am a true believer in my spiritual world, even though this may not fit in with other people's beliefs, I am a part of God, and this is where my inner strength comes from. This is not a religious belief, it is a human belief that we all have an inner power – the power that lives while we do, the power that keeps us coming back for more.

This means when you're working with children, it may help you to find out for yourself what your centre is and to explore what you're likely to find if you were to ask these questions:

What do you think your centre is?

What does it mean?

What does it represent for you?

How much of your everyday life is affected by your centre?

These are deep questions for many people. Some have deep religious faith so this can be part of their centres. Others may not be able to pinpoint it so easily and perhaps think all their life experiences and beliefs simply come from their consciousness.

However, I believe our centre is the deepest part of ourselves that makes us human and that it's an area few of us have explored.

To be able to live from our centres means we can be more balanced and emotionally well.

Whatever it is that has given me the chance to experience the life I have led, is also part of my true self – the one I want to be true to, to be the best I can, every day of this life I am privileged to have. It is the place where the real Rene resides – the one I am proud of and, when it's all over, I know I have done the best I possibly can.

I tell children who I work with, and sometimes adults who need to learn this, the centre is the place where they can always feel okay within themselves. I tell them this is the place where they can find their strengths, their own ideas of what they want to do and believe in to make them strong and brave.

I tried to teach my granddaughters, and now my grandson, this aspect of my beliefs, especially when they have been emotionally drawn into the events in other people's lives. For example, Dakota was always very emotionally attached to her mother and half-brothers. When she decided to let go and not be drawn into the drama of their lives which happened each time she had contact, she was able to make adult decisions, to let go, and get on with her own life.

So, as I work with children, I refer to their centres, their hearts and their loves and, in this way, it becomes part of their everyday lives.

I hope, through this teaching, the child can develop a better sense of self. I also believe that this helps children develop character traits they can carry with them through to their adult lives.

This is not an easy aspect of emotional intelligence to work with as it engages deeply personal issues for both parent and child. Patience is necessary here because children will often close up when you talk about these aspects of their character and how they deal with them. However, I included this section in my book because I found it to be an important part of my own emotional growth, and perhaps others reading this will too.

Understanding emotions is an integral part of my work and this book. For many people, it is sometimes easier to push their emotions down and deny having any at all. For others, the feelings may nag away until the person does get 'real' and tries to understand just what is happening in their emotional life that's affecting other aspects of their life. They may wonder why they always feel so tired and have no energy. They may ask themselves *Why do I think I miss out all the time and why doesn't anybody listen to me?*

I worked with a lass a few months ago who had no understanding of emotions. She had no words for what they actually were – no emotional vocabulary. She also had no understanding of what I was trying to tell her, nor any point of reference.

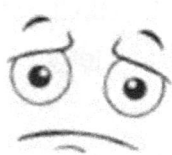

WHAT ARE EMOTIONS?

An emotion is an energy that occurs when we have an interaction with the outside world. It is the resulting feeling we get when something happens in our lives. Emotions are temporary, because they come and go. They pass through us, and as we allow ourselves to acknowledge them and feel them, they will move on and leave space for the next emotion.

At times, we allow them to take control of our lives and this makes it difficult to understand exactly what is happening to us.

For some people, emotions can bring illness and disease, yet some people still can't understand what's happening because they don't acknowledge the emotion that exists.

Many of us grew up in homes where our parents didn't teach us about dealing with our emotions, because they were never taught how to deal with theirs. Please know, there is no blame meant here – this is just the reality that happened to people who dearly loved their children.

As we grew up, we went to school where emotions were not part of the school curriculum. Thank goodness that is slowly changing as schools today are beginning to realise the value of incorporating emotional intelligence into the curriculum.

As these issues were not addressed at all years ago, we continued to develop into teenagers, with the inevitable emotional and hormonal changes happening to us all, and our feelings were still not dealt with. As a result, no-one actually understood what was happening to them, or to their peers.

When we grew to adulthood, many of us fell in love and this hit many of us hard. For many, this was the fairytale come true and their lives were settled and happy. Yet for many others, the fairytale did not eventuate and their lives were anything but happy. Often these people had no idea the extent to which their unrecognised emotions were ruining their lives. These people had no idea how to read, understand, or to work with their emotions to make their lives happier and less stressful.

It's important to remember that our emotions move through us. You can see a great example of this when you watch a small child at play and see how quickly the emotions pass through them. I have observed many little ones and I have seen the quick changes that happen – the laughter as the car runs up the sandhill, the frustration when the car gets bogged, the sadness when they cannot get it to move, and the absolute joy when they succeed in moving this car on.

And this is what happens with us, as adults. There are many names for the emotions we feel each and every day – happy, sad, pissed off, stressed, scared, excited, grief stricken, frustrated, and so the list goes on.

Ask yourself: *How many emotions can I write down in a minute; how many do I feel each day; what is the emotion I feel the most and do I acknowledge it? If not, why not?*

In my work as a counsellor and facilitator, I classify the emotions into five groups, and for me these five groups include every emotion we feel. All emotions are just energy which means they are all okay as they are neither negative nor positive.

JOY

Joy is the energy of receiving and connecting. What is it that makes us feel happy and filled with joy? What does this emotion feel like? Where do we feel it? I feel it in my whole body, especially in my heart as it feels as if it is full and overflowing. I feel lighter on the earth, I smile at people I don't even know, and they smile back. I want to laugh and sing, and so I do. I do stupid things that others are often appalled at, like not always smiling in photos, and my crazy impulses get me into awful strife.

I am filled with love for other people and I would like to show this by giving them a hug – by dancing, laughing and having a wonderful time.

I also feel joy when I am on my own and walking – in the forest or by the sea, where there is a peacefulness and a knowledge that all is right with my world.

I feel joy when I have completed a job, or an application for a job and a chapter of a new book. I sometimes even feel joy when I have washed the floor and done the dishes, so the sink is clean and uncluttered. I remember feeling joy when I hung snow white nappies on the line to dry. I feel great when I have completed a tai chi class and I know my students have learned something new and have enjoyed a peaceful hour where they've been able to relax and learn.

I love it when I spend time with my grandchildren and know they are happy in my home.

Happiness, joy and love are all tied up with this emotion.

Children love this emotion as they are naturally exuberant and mostly filled with love and sunshine. We all live to succeed, and children laugh when they are having fun, loving their lives and just being kids.

As adults we sometimes forget that this happiness can be ours any time we want. We just have to allow it to happen.

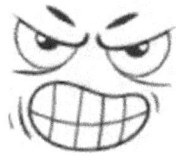

ANGER

What is anger?

We all have a different interpretation of what anger is but I believe it's how we deal with it that gives us the answer.

For me, anger is an energy that is created when my boundaries are threatened; when something I love or cherish is in danger of being taken away from me; when my ideas and actions are not accepted but rejected; when I am busy doing something and my granddaughter rings me to tell me she is almost home and asks to be picked up, interrupting my time and energy.

This can be a fleeting spurt of anger, or it can be a slow burning that needs to be dealt with as soon as possible.

Anger is the most feared emotion in our society today as there is so much violence, or threat of violence, with actions fuelled by rage impacting communities.

For me, rage is anger that has not been dealt with early enough to stop it becoming worse. It has been allowed to fester and grow – it has no way out and therefore it builds up inside so that the resulting violence is anger's way of expressing itself. It is allowed to get out of control and therefore it holds great power.

Sadly, some of our children are raised in houses and countries where rage and hatred run hand in hand. Parents who cannot control their own anger take it out on the people around them and someone always gets hurt.

For the purposes of this book, I will only refer to anger as an energy in our everyday lives and in our children's lives.

Emotions that make up anger include irritation, frustration, being 'pissed off', feeling upset and needing to yell.

Children often feel anger in their everyday lives: when they can't get their own way; as new siblings arrive; as they grow up and life presents them with challenges. Each child reacts in a different way and mum is usually the person this anger is directed at.

Children can be shown how to deal with anger safely, rather than pushing it away and storing it. Each parent and carer can work out which is the safest and best way for their child to let go of their anger.

Some children are very quiet and timid, yet still feel anger so, for them, yelling may not be appropriate. You need to find a physical way to help these kids, such as giving them a bat and ball, challenging them to yell and throw.

It's important for you to find a way to work with your child that suits you both. Perhaps singing some songs together, cutting and pasting while talking, or throwing water at each other.

FEAR

Fear is the energy we feel when we lose someone or something we love.

There are two types of fear:

Real fear is when we know we are in danger of being hurt or annihilated, for example in cases of an earthquake, a tsunami, a bomb attack – events we have no control over and that will certainly cause us physical suffering. The best way to deal with this fear is to breathe deeply and face what is going to happen, or, alternatively, make it to a safe place!

Mind-generated fear is where our minds play out 'videos' and show us scenarios that we fear might happen. These images are only in our minds and there is no guarantee they will happen at all, but still we worry and stress – *What if I don't have enough money to pay my home loan?* The bank will repossess the house and we'll be homeless. *What will happen to my kids?* We will be thrown out on the streets and we'll starve!" And so the dialogue continues.

Often, a small thought can generate a huge amount of fear. Children have these mind-generated fears too so don't dismiss them. Listen and help where you can.

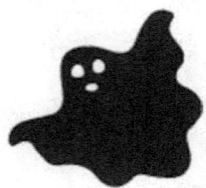

Recently, my eight-year-old grandson didn't want to go to sleep because he thought there were killer clowns around, and they might come into our house. So, I talked to him about the realness of this happening and introduced the idea that his mind was making up these stories and they were not real. We talked about it for a while and he was happy enough to see that his mind was playing games with him and went off to sleep. I didn't use the term 'mind-generated' as he's too young. I just said his mind was making up stories and he could choose whether or not to believe them.

Children can be so easily helped and their fears allayed when a parent assists the child to find the truth and understand the 'games' our minds play on us, as well as the reasons for this fear.

When I headed off to China for a year to teach English, many people told me how brave I was. Yet I had deep fears about going and they seemed to be very real. One day, I found myself lost in the bush. I was in an unknown place, just on dark, and no one knew where I was. I did not know which way to go. As I had learned skills to cope with fear, I asked myself what I needed to do to find the way out. I thought hard and eventually I did make my way out of the bush. This experience taught me a huge lesson. One day before I left for China, I sat down and thought through the fears that I had about going and allowed myself to feel scared and lost. I then allowed these feelings to slip away as I found the answers that I needed. I knew I had the courage – I had a job to go to, I would be met at the plane by delegates from the university, I would be housed and fed, and I was earning money. I was also very excited about the whole experience as it presented an adventure. During this period in my life, I found that fear and being nervous is sometimes part of excitement. We just need to feel it and work out what it represents.

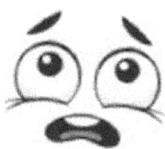

During the whole time I was in China, I only ever felt fear twice. This was because I wasn't sure what was going to happen to me and I was on my own, in an uncertain situation. However, in the end, it all actually worked out okay.

Children's fears need to be vocalised. My grandson used to be afraid of the huge electric structures that dominate parts of our landscape. Both his parents and I explained to him that they were steel structures to carry power to all of the people. While writing this, I think it could have also been good to walk him towards one and allow him to feel the steel.

Sometimes a child will vocalise a fear and it's very important to honour that fear and not put them down or laugh at them. Explain to them the best you can, look it up in a reference book, or perhaps 'Google it', helping them see the truth for themselves. It may not totally erase the fear but the truth is there for the child to examine for themselves.

Sometimes with my young adult clients I have asked them to ask themselves – *What is the worst that can happen and how would you feel?*

Thinking about this question has given them the opportunity to step back and look again. I had a young lady I was helping whose sight was fading so her fear was real. By asking her to face what might happen she was able to choose some answers for herself and prepare the way for the future – also by facing this, she was able to stay in the present.

Fear can be a terrifying feeling for us as adults, but for children it's sometimes overwhelming. This is when the adult needs to be able to remain calm and help the child to understand just what is happening. If it is real fear, then it's important the adult stays as in control as possible. If it is mind-generated, then the parent needs to be able to explain to the child just what their mind and imagination is manifesting.

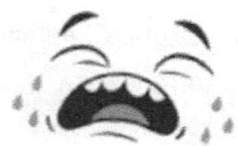

SADNESS

Sadness is the energy of loss – the feeling we have when we lose something or someone we love and value. For many years I hid my sadness with anger as it was easier to do this. My sadness would have crippled me at this time, so I worked a way to hide it. Sadness was not an emotion I wanted to be associated with. Anger, on the other hand, was an energy I could use to fuel my life.

I had experienced a broken marriage, ended by me as I left and took the three boys with me.

When this happened, I had to change all the plans I had made, which was to rear my boys while I stayed at home and to go back to full time work, when I was ready. Becoming a single parent meant my boys would sometimes have to come home to a house without me in it, and I had to become the sole breadwinner, meaning I was often tired and angry.

Above all of this I felt I had failed, so I hid my failure, my feelings of abandonment, my fears of not being strong enough to do this, with anger. At the time, I had no idea what the boys were feeling, or how they were coping without their father and with a full-time working mother. I just went ahead and brought them up the best way I could.

My mother added to this mix by ringing me every night and telling me, how terrible I was, what an awful mother I was and how dare I take my boys away from their father. Now I understand she must have been terribly worried, not knowing if I could cope, and, being 'old school', she must have thought, how could I leave their father? So, for me, I think the sadness got so buried, I never really saw it as that. I was just angry with the world. Underneath it all, was this terrible guilt, this feeling I had let everybody down.

Many years later, I watched the girls' sadness turn into anger – anger with their parents and probably with me, for discouraging them from returning to their parents. In later years, I saw their sadness turn into detachment when they realised that whatever they did, their parents would not step in and take them – they would not change.

Sadness, grief, disappointment and all that entails, causes deep scars in the soul of a child and many repress these feelings – gloss over them, make them less real, in order to not feel the pain.

Scratch the surface of a child who lives out of home care and you will find there are a myriad of feelings under there that need to be acknowledged, and hopefully dealt with.

A little child will cry when they are sad. When nobody comes to help them understand how to let go of this feeling, it goes deep inside and they bury it so they don't have to feel the pain. They manage to hide it and, as a result, often react with anger, sometimes violence.

Bullying is sometimes a cover for deep sadness, so it's important to deal with the bully, as well as with the bullied, and find out what causes there are for this behaviour.

When my youngest son, Nick, was in his first year at school, he was being bullied every day, by one of the older boys. Nick was a sensitive child and this boy had worked out how to upset him and make him cry. When the situation was eventually resolved, it turned out the older boy smelled. This was not his fault, but he was ostracised by his classmates as a result and took his sadness and anger out on Nick. Fortunately, the school principal at the time believed in getting to the bottom of these types of situations and this boy was helped. For me, this was an important lesson in the importance of looking past the obvious to find out just why anger is there.

APATHY, EMPTINESS AND NOTHINGNESS

Not being able to feel any emotions, or give them a name is often a form of not caring – an inability to understand reactions to what is happening around you. I have called this section 'Apathy', for want of a better word. It is when we don't understand or care what's happening inside us and take no responsibility for our reactions to everyday events, nor value the lessons we learn along the way.

Many people don't know how to react when things happen in their lives. Sometimes overwhelming events happen in life and the person pushes the feelings down because they are too strong and too scary. It's safer to not acknowledge them and allow them to have any meaning in their lives. It doesn't always mean that they don't care. It just means they are unaware of the importance of owning their feelings and allowing them credence in their everyday lives.

Some people who have had difficult childhoods – perhaps they have grown up with violent parents, been abused in some way, or been treated with disrespect – may choose to push their feelings down so they're not experiencing pain any more. It may sometimes explain the unacceptable anger they demonstrate in daily life, the nasty way they treat other people and the unhappiness inside.

These people may have shown their emotions in the past and been put down or experienced a bad reaction from the people around them. As a result, they have pushed their emotions down as deeply as they can, so they don't have to suffer any more. Because these people, in the past, have learned to suppress their feelings, they feel nothing and admit to nothing.

When I worked in China, I was very aware of the special place I held within this university. I was the only native English-speaking person on a campus of five thousand students, many teachers and external staff. I was proud to be Australian so I decided I needed to be even-tempered and gracious at all times, even though there were occasions when I felt I could have exploded and expressed how I truly felt. Of course, there were things that happened and brought up emotions for me. For example, when I was left out of discussions about what I was supposed to teach and told to just "talk to students". The frustration when I couldn't have access to a telephone to phone home and couldn't open my door on hot nights. For nearly a year I kept these emotions in check which was not really doing myself any good as there were times when I was incredibly lonely and longed for an Australian voice, or was able to have a good yell and vent. When I finally arrived home, I attended a weekend workshop where I was able to let it all go.

Children are the same as adults in this respect. If they don't feel safe expressing themselves, they tend to bottle up all their feelings. When they are given the opportunity to let their feelings out, in a safe environment, the emotions will all be released and your child will feel better.

Summer was very good at hiding her feelings because she learned, very early in her life, that it was not acceptable to her mother so she pushed all her emotions down and this has continued to affect her.

It is not good for anyone to push down their feelings and ignore them. This can affect how well we sleep, eat, cause disease and result in a lack of honesty.

I referred earlier to the work I did with Master Life Coach, Nicholas de Castella and, with his permission, I have included his teachings on what he refers to as 'Head and Heart Distinctions':

Thinking: The mind/head/brain.
Aspects: Thoughts, beliefs, assumptions, judgements, guilt, shame.
Processes: Memory, imagination, calculations, planning, deduction, manipulation, analysis.
Comparisons: Generalisations, sort, judge, inspiration.
Functions: Linear, logical, rational, based on past patterning and paradigms.

Feeling: The heart/body.
Qualities: Love, care, compassion, gratitude, appreciation, security, patience, forgiveness.
Functions as: Feeling, intuition, flowing energy, animation, sincerity, authenticity, responsive to the moment.

Emotions: Energy created in our interaction with the outside world. Emotions are temporary as they come and go. As we allow ourselves to feel them, they will move on and leave a space for the next emotion – a great example of this is to watch a small child at play and see how quickly the emotions pass through.

I group emotions together in five groups, and for me, all emotions fall into one or other of these groups:

Joy – The energy of receiving and connecting.

Sadness – The energy of loss – when we lose something or someone we want or value.

Fear – The energy of looking like we are going to lose something/someone we love.

Anger – The energy created when our boundaries are threatened.

Nothing – When we don't let ourselves really care what we get or want or value, or we are so used to being unemotional we don't feel anything.

> "If we are to teach real peace in this world, and if we are to carry on a real war against war, we shall have to begin with the children."
>
> — MAHATMA GANDHI

> "Pretty much all the honest truth telling there is in the world is done by children."

OLIVER WENDELL HOLMES

CHAPTER 7
Dealing With Toxic Shame

What is shame?

What part does it play in the story of our emotions?

How can I help my child deal with this type of shame?

Doctor Jo Horwood, my local GP for many years and a 'Deep Field Relaxation' practitioner, wrote an article once called 'How Shame Makes us Sick.'[1] This was based on an article by Nicholas de Castella, 'The Anatomy of Shame.'[2] I have based this chapter on the combined work Nicholas and Jo have done in this area.

Shame is an e-motion – energy in motion.

It can be healthy or unhealthy. **Healthy shame** is the feeling we get when we make a mistake, the purpose of which is to remind us of our essential humanity – that we can make mistakes and often do. We can then apologise, learn from the mistake and change our actions next time this situation occurs – "I have made the mistake, but I'm still okay".

Unhealthy or toxic shame is the feeling of sadness in which we feel we are wrong, bad or invalid. Toxic shame says, "I am a mistake".

WHAT IS SHAME?

According to the online free dictionary, Wikipedia, "shame is a negative, painful, social emotion, caused by the awareness of doing something wrong."

Therapy books suggest shame comes from being taught that we are worthless, bad, or something similar.

So, why do I include a discussion of shame in my book?

I have included this topic in my book as I believe children are sometimes shamed at home, even though it may not be the intention of the person doing the shaming.

Some time ago, I had a father as a client who was being shamed by his wife. It had seriously dented his self-esteem, so much so he had allowed himself to become a victim. When he was feeling particularly down, he would yell at his little children because he couldn't see another way to do this in the space he was in; "Shut up, you're too loud! Why don't you do it this way! You're a little s... head!"

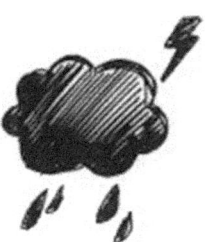

In his moments of clarity, he would never let this happen, but his wife's shaming and his lack of self-esteem dragged him down. Unless he did a lot of work on his own self-confidence, his children would continue to suffer.

For me, and from what I have observed in some of my clients, I think shaming fits into certain aspects of sadness, as it is not always an angry emotion, nor is it fearful or joyful. It reflects sadness and disappointment – "I have done wrong; I am not good enough; I have made a mistake; I do not live up to people's expectations; I am not a good provider, and for all of that, I will be judged. I will pay a price I should not have to".

If I have done something wrong there should be a consequence, when there is no resulting consequence there may be a feeling of shame.

My mother made me feel wrong many times in my life because I didn't fulfil her dreams of how her daughter should be. I had two sisters and I was certainly different from them. However, for my mother, I was not as good as my sisters. She called me "stupid" and thought I was wrong when I left my husband, even though he had physically assaulted me – "You must have done something wrong for that to happen," were her words.

So, for many years I felt the shame of knowing I had failed her and, therefore, I was not good enough. After years of working with emotions I know now that it was her problem, not mine. She did not understand what 'made me tick' and she was probably very fearful of how I could be hurt.

In my classrooms I only made one rule – no put downs, which meant accepting others, including their comments, ideas and answers. It also meant no laughing or judging others and allowing them to have a different outlook and energy to mine. We are all here to learn and our ideas, though different, are all acceptable, and it also brings out the best in people if they can accept and consider the ideas of others. Children are so easily shamed – they speak from their ideas, from their hearts, they think they're right even when they're not. They need to be able to test their thoughts with others and be encouraged to share their ideas about the world around them. We, as parents and carers, need to know how to listen and to hear what they're saying, or trying to say, with honour and without judgement.

Shame occurs when a child or a person puts forward an idea that is not accepted by the listener. The listener might laugh or scoff and put aside the idea being presented as being ridiculous or not acceptable. Sometimes, children have fantastic ideas as their imaginations take flight and they often come up with stories, ideas and things they believe are acceptable, even though to adults they're unrealistic. It can be hard for a parent to seriously listen to a far-out suggestion with patience and help the child realise its inadequacies, rather than putting it down straight away, calling it stupid.

I have such an aversion to the word 'stupid' and I realise it's because of the incident with my mother when she used this word multiple times, during a twenty-minute tirade, when I told her I had taken a year off teaching to complete my second degree.

This is the time to work out your priorities. If your child tells you a fantastic story, hear it out and consider it before answering and, either deflate their ego, or stoke it sensibly. The child's heart is all in the things they create, and, if shamed, even though they may be too young to understand what the word means, they do know anger, frustration and sadness. I also see children taking this one step further and this is what we have to guard against – the child may take out their frustration on another child or a younger sibling and this needs to stop.

As a parent or carer, it's important to sometimes stop and listen to what your child says to other children and how they say it. Does it sound like you? Is he repeating what you say?

Is this what you want to hear? How can you change it so your child will become less shamed?

Here are some ideas and ways to help your child deal with feelings of shame, based on the work of Doctor Jo Horwood who stresses the importance of finding, 'a place where we can break the spell of silence about our shame, talk about it and know we are safe'. Find a safe place and talk to someone who is non-judgemental and caring, who will listen to what you have to say and not try to fix it.

According to Dr Horwood, "a safe place is where we can break the spell of silence about our shame, talk about it and know we will be safe." A child may cover their feelings of shame with anger or sadness, and it's up to you, as their carer, to uncover these feelings they are hiding.

I felt a lot of shame in my younger years as I was loud and didn't conform to the standards set by my sisters, who probably never knew I felt like this. My mother often reminded me I was not as good as my sisters, in many ways, so I took this shame into my adulthood. Talking with one of my sisters about this once, she said that she had also felt shamed, so perhaps my mother used this strategy to get her message across.

Stop shaming yourself and others. Learn to recognise the ways in which we shame and take steps to correct them.

In the language we use with our children, it's very important to be aware of the effect our words have on them. For example, with today's fashion of low-waisted jeans, short shorts and plenty of bare skin showing, it's easy to be critical. However, we need to remember that little girls love to emulate older girls in the way they dress. Even if you don't approve of the outfit, be very careful how you frame your comment and make sure it's positive criticism, not shaming. Fashions will change, and little girls need the chance to test out their own dress sense.

Stand up for your rights and teach your child how to do this. If you learn about assertiveness, which involves respecting your own rights, your own sense of self-worth grows and you also learn to respect the rights of others.

Ask your child to consider the following:

What are my rights?

What do I want to be respected for in my life?

What is causing me to feel shame because this respect is not happening?

Try to learn about assertiveness and teach your child what it is, and how to use it in a respectful way. In this way, you will learn to develop your own self-respect and be more likely to value and defend the rights of others.

In today's world, I believe girls in particular, should be taught they do have rights and how to stand up for them. There are many countries in the world where females have no rights – where they are abused and treated as second class citizens. As a result, they end up believing they're not worthwhile and go through life without being honoured as individuals.

Teaching our little boys how to treat a woman with respect is also long overdue, and that lesson should start at home. For little boys, it is equally important they learn about their own personal rights, how to be caring and proud in this world, whilst respecting the rights of others, especially their mothers and sisters.

Teaching fathers to value and respect themselves is also very important because how can a father make sure his little girl is treated with the respect she deserves, if he doesn't respect himself?

If we teach our children assertiveness, which involves respect for yourself, they grow as a person and also learn respect for the rights of others. When boundaries are disrespected a child needs to be able to stand up for themselves and know they are acceptable in this world. A parent can teach a child how to respect themselves by providing love and care, as well as positive feedback and constructive criticism.

My firm belief has always been that, if I expect a child to respect me, then I must show the child respect first. This always worked for me as a teacher and as a friend. It's important to help a child learn about self-respect and this will lead into respect for others and standing up for their rights.

It's okay to experience shame when you have made a mistake, as long as it's clear that **you are not the mistake.**

Common areas in life where we may be shamed include:

Our bodies: are too thin, too fat, wrong shaped nose, big teeth, too tall or too short.

Our feelings: are too emotional, too loud, too soft, a 'sooky baby', 'grizzle guts'.

Our minds: stupid ideas, "how could you be so stupid?", "get real, grow up".

Our sexuality: "cover yourself up", "you look like a tart", "stop playing with yourself, if you masturbate you'll go blind."

Everyone needs a sense of shame, but no-one needs to feel ashamed.

WAYS TO ENHANCE A CHILD'S SELF-ESTEEM

I include the following ideas for helping children build their self-esteem. I believe it's an important gift we can give our children to help them feel good about themselves. While you work with your child, perhaps you may also find your own self-esteem improves.

Have photos of the child framed and displayed about the house. In my grandchildren's bedrooms they have framed baby photos, photos of them with parents and friends. These are ongoing and added to as the years pass. In this way, the child can see they are loved and are important enough to be put 'on show'.

Put the photo albums where they can be reached and share time with your child browsing through them. Talk about how beautiful they were and still are and how much they are loved. Share stories about the times shown in the photos.

As they go through kindergarten and school, and bring home the work they have done, put it up where it can be seen – usually on the fridge, so it can be seen and admired. Afterwards, it can be used in a variety of ways: put it together as a book; use it as wrapping paper for presents; as wallpaper in a cubby house; photo frames for grandparents' gifts – any way where the child sees that what he has done is acceptable, honoured and useful. I know that when you have more than one child this can become difficult but with thought and imagination, you can always find creative and thoughtful ways to use these creations. For example, grandparents are often happy to take and display some of the work when you've run out of fridge and wall space.

Give your child a photo album that is theirs to keep and they can add to it as they wish. Provide photos that show who the child really is. Ideally, these photos should represent the many people in your child's life so they can see they are loved and accepted by a variety of people.

Introduce the ideas of self-responsibility to your child. For example, encourage your child to take responsibility for their self-care, say things like – "Now you are big enough you might like to help me keep your room tidy, make your bed and brush your own hair." Praise them for things they have done as this will help the child grow.

When a new baby arrives, an older child can help the parent by getting nappies when change time happens. Setting the table is a great activity as it helps reinforce simple mathematical concepts, and being given this responsibility will give the child a feeling of usefulness – "I am an important member of this family." These simple jobs can lead to other chores as the child gets older.

Talk with your child about the concept of cause and effect in behaviour – If something goes wrong discuss with the child what happened and ask them, "What else could you have done to change the outcome of this?" Listen to and acknowledge their answer.

Some time ago my grandson was most upset as one of the boys at his kindergarten called him mean and this hurt his feelings. He was pushing his friend on the swing when the boy fell off and hurt himself. One of the other children saw this happen and called my grandson mean, which worried him. His dad talked to him, asked him what had happened, listened and then asked what he felt about it. He replied that he could see that it was an accident and accepted he was not being mean.

Allow children to select their own clothes and dress themselves. When appropriateness needs to be considered, help the child choose what can be worn and comment positively so their own sense of colour and style can be developed. It also helps them understand that saying **' no'** is okay.

Thank your child for what they do and give – "Nan, your hair looks lovely! Thank you!" Children then learn to make other positive comments when they know they are heard.

Introduce your child to their breathing. This vital aspect of our lives is often taken for granted and young children can be taught to feel and listen to their own breath.

Once a day, encourage your child to stand or sit still, close their eyes and feel their breath. I place one hand on their middle back and the other on their tummy, ask them to close their eyes and breathe. With some children it takes a little longer to overcome the giggles, but if you persevere it becomes a few moments of inner peace for them.

Our breath is our lifeline to mental, emotional and physical balance and if we can help children to become aware of their breathing they will also learn about the power of the breath.

AFFIRMATIONS FOR YOUR PRESCHOOLER (NICHOLAS DE CASTELLA)

I love watching you grow.

I will be here for you to test your boundaries and find out your limits.

It's okay for you to think about yourself.

You can think about your feelings and have
feelings about what you are thinking.

I like your life energy.

I like your curiosity about sex — (sometimes
very confronting for parents) .

It's okay to find out the difference between boys and girls.

I will set limits for you to help you find out who you are.

I like it that you are a boy/girl.

It's okay to cry, even though you're growing up.

It's okay to feel angry, sad and fearful.

You can ask for what you want.

You can ask questions if something confuses you.

You are not responsible for your mum.

You are not responsible for your dad.

It's okay to explore who you are.

AFFIRMATIONS FOR YOUR TEENAGER

I love your life energy.

I love who you are.

I love watching you make decisions for yourself.

I love the way you embrace life and make your own decisions.

I love the way you question my rules.

I love the way you push the boundaries yet stop
when you know you have gone too far.

I love the way you talk with me and share your dreams.

I love to see you dressed up ready to go out and
your expectations of what will happen.

I love how you ask for explanations about drugs, alcohol and sex.

I love you just as you are.

I also love how you accept me as me –
just as I am, no holds barred.

I also love how you 'crack the sads' and go to your
room, as I know that this the dance of life, and
you will get over it and come out smiling.

I love your expectations and your fears for the
future – sharing your ideas and plans for the future
is sacred to me and I honour the sharing.

I love to use the words, "tears are welcome here".

BOUNDARIES – WHAT ARE THEY?

Boundaries are all about our personal space, both physical and emotional.

Just how close do I want a person to stand near me, or I want to stand near them?

Do I want a person to touch me or not?

Where do I want them to touch me?

Do I want to be hugged?

Do I want to change my clothes in a quiet space and have no one see me?

How close can I let a person near me before I feel threatened?

Are there certain places on my body I do not want touched?

How often do I need time alone?

What will I allow others to do for me?

And there are countless more boundaries, which will differ for all of us, so you need to consider what matters to you.

I hate being touched by strangers and, sometimes in a room full of people, I have to leave as I feel I don't have enough physical space. This is my way of keeping myself safe.

I also need time every day to be myself – to be able to do what it is I want to do, read a book, watch a show, walk in the garden, just a little time for me.

Setting your own boundaries is also crucial in a relationship so people understand your boundaries, or feel they can ask if it's not clear. It helps people better understand what their partners want in the relationship and what they're willing to share with each other. When a family can set their own boundaries through discussion – I don't want you to go through my purse, for example – and discuss the implications, they're better able to support each other and respect individual boundaries.

Everybody has boundaries. Think about your own.

> *How do you express to others what your boundaries are and how you would like them respected?*
>
> *How much do you allow other people to influence your life?*
>
> *Have you set your boundaries clearly in your relationships?*
>
> *How do you feel when they are disrespected?*

When you understand your own boundaries, you can then talk with your child and introduce the ideas of boundaries – for them and for others. This discussion can also bring in the important issue of sexual and physical boundaries – what the child can do if these are violated, such as who to tell.

One of my young friends does not like anyone to touch her in the back of the neck – she has no idea why, but she has made this very clear to her family and friends so we don't touch her there.

Healthy boundaries are when a child can regulate their reality and use their own energy to set and enhance their boundaries, as well as to learn to respect other people's boundaries.

Encourage your child to verbalise this and say what they want and what they don't want.

Avoid long explanations – a child's interest is lost very quickly and much can be expressed in fewer words.

Be honest with your own feelings – children may become fearful when a parent cries or yells, but if you explain how you're feeling and that this is the way you are able to express it, you can reassure the child.

If you feel the fear is too great, use the 'sounding' in the shower method – using your voice, make a sound as deep in your throat as you possibly can, holding it as long as you're able.

When the girls were little and still emotionally fragile, I used this method to move the angry/fearful energy within me. It always ended up in tears but that was good.

Honour your child's feelings and responses and accept them as they express them, letting them know it's okay to feel sad or angry.

Nicholas de Castella teaches that "honouring is a word used to describe the act of really hearing, feeling and responding to others in a way that is respectful, validating, empathetic and deeply loving".

Three steps of honouring you can share with your child in response to their emotional expression are:

ACKNOWLEDGEMENT

Sit down with the child in a quiet place where you are unlikely to be interrupted and listen intently. Be very present with what the child says and don't allow your own thoughts to interrupt the flow of words and thoughts – especially if you don't agree or feel you know better. The child has the right to be heard. Be fully present with them and maintain eye contact. Be able to feed back to them exactly what they said – "I hear that you are feeling sad because I yelled at you."

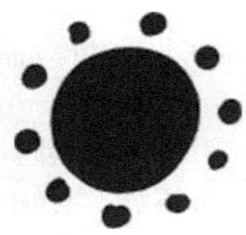

VALIDATION AND UNDERSTANDING

Be understanding and imagine you are in their place and try to relate to similar experiences in your life, without taking over. "I understand you feel sad because I yelled at you. I can remember feeling sad when my mum yelled at me".

EMPATHISE

Give a response from your heart. Share how you feel and what emotions you're experiencing as a result of what they have shared with you. To do this, we need to let the sharing come in and touch us by opening our hearts. Sometimes, we have to put our own feelings aside and once the child feels honoured you can then express your own feelings – "I feel really sad that you felt so sad when I yelled and I will really make an effort to not yell at you. Then, if I sometimes forget and do this, you can remind me of what I have said."

Be very aware that you do not make the child feel wrong in their feelings. It just has to be a comment to validate the child and show that you have heard them. Also be careful that you're not asking the child to make your feelings right – these feelings need to be owned by the speaker and heard by the listener, not taken on by either one.

CHAMPIONING FEELINGS

If the child does not feel honoured by you when they share, help them to learn to stand up for their feelings. To do this, a child needs to understand that the feeling they have is okay and they don't need you to fix it, only to hear it and validate it. It can be a difficult concept for a small child, but as the child grows within this relationship with you, so will their understanding.

Honouring is the opposite of shaming. Shaming dismisses, invalidates and blocks our emotions. Honouring acknowledges, validates and supports the truth of our being.

When we, as parents and carers, honour our children, they feel loved by us and then, as they begin to honour us, we can feel loved by them. Honouring is also a gift we can give ourselves by trusting our own experiences and for standing up for what we believe and feel to be true.

For some parents the whole idea of honouring may be new and a bit scary. As children, many of us were not encouraged to speak our truths, much less say how we really felt. In many homes, children were 'seen and not heard' and it was very rare for a child to have their point of views listened to.

You may have grown up hearing comments like: "Go to your room! Who wants to listen to you?! Shut up! What would you know – you're just a kid!"

However, probably as an indirect result of our need to be heard, and our need to feel valued, many of us have changed our ways of thinking and look for other ways of being with our children.

Children today do not want to be not seen and not heard!

From an early age children are vocal and self-opinionated, they learn their rights very quickly and sometimes tell us very loudly they want to be heard and, as carers of our children, we have choices:

We can allow the child to be as vocal and as loud as they wish.

We can 'crush' the child and allow no self-expression.

We can explore our own feelings and begin to make the changes in our lives so our child can explore their own feelings, try out their own ideas, learn to speak out loud, be heard and learn to live with their own truth.

It takes great courage and persistence for a parent to walk this path as many of these issues may be confronting and challenge a parent's own values. Sometimes it's essential for the parent to do some work on themselves before they're able to help their children grow in faith and honesty.

Consider this. There's a great difference between a child who's well fed, well dressed and well educated, yet feels as though they're not loved, to a child who has grown within the boundaries of love and validation, who will enter the world with more confidence, hope and self-esteem.

According to Nicholas de Castella, children are put down and invalidated when they hear these comments or witness these types of behaviour:

A parent is angry with a child, or feels that they are at war with them, the adult attacks the child with/by personal criticism.

"You look like a tart in that outfit." – Personal criticism

"You broke the bottle didn't you!" – Accusations

"What makes you think you know it all?" – Sarcasm

"You are just like your mother." – Generalising

"P… off, let me do it." – Dismissive comments, swearing and shouting

"What a stupid idea! Wherever did you get such a stupid idea from?" – Mean comments

"Why can't you be more like your sister?" – Comparisons

"Get over here now!" – Sharp and abrupt comments

Cold shouldering and not talking – Creating insecurity

Running late to pick them up/drop them off – Your child is not a priority.

"Do it yourself!" – Refusing to help

The tones used in these messages also give the child fair warning of what the adult is saying and, when accompanied by aggressive, angry body behaviour, a child **knows** they are being put down.

In response, the child will often become defensive by:

- **Running away or perhaps hiding and taking themselves out of the line of parental activity.**
  - Being quiet and 'invisible' – watching television or hiding with their iPad.
  - Being pleasing, becoming the 'polite' child outside the home, who doesn't answer back, who behaves nicely all of the time, but at home is the opposite.
  - Excessive apologising for things they may not have done but feel they have to do this to keep in the good books.
  - Physical withdrawal – where they take themselves off to a separate place.

- **Emotional withdrawal – where they will not talk to you or answer your questions.**
  - Excuse making – finding reasons why they can't be available when their parent(s) want them to be.
  - Rebellion – fighting against everything and anything.
  - Justification – feeling they have the right to be where they are and not answer to their parent(s).

- Explanations – excessive explaining about what they have done and why.
- Extremely good, followed by bad behaviour.
- Crying easily.
- Being insolent.

Never underestimate a child's feelings or ability to understand a situation. A 'mistake' is when I get an outcome I don't expect so it's always a learning experience. An original is better than a copy any day.

I remember times in my life when I used some of these negative tones in the messages I gave to my children – times when I was tired and angry and didn't feel like being thoughtful and considerate. As the saying goes, "shit happens!" We are parents and there are a myriad of things happening in our lives, every day, that cause pain and worry. However, for most parents, these negative messages to our children are the exception rather than the norm, so don't beat yourself up when a slip happens. Apologise to your child and get on with what really matters.

It's important to always be aware of differences in children within families – what works for one may not always work for another.

When I was working with two sisters whose family background was fraught with violence and nastiness, I found it a challenge as both girls were extremely emotionally damaged. Their responses and their needs were very different so I needed to tread very carefully and not confuse the differences I observed between these two girls.

For the first few visits, the older girl would hide in the hole under my writing desk, telling me that this was where she felt the safest. As I gained her trust, she became more vocal, yet I sensed a certain reticence to really 'let go'. So, one day I talked with her about angels and how we could have them as our support if we simply asked. I suggested it was a safe place in my house to let go and the angels would take the pain and the anger away if she would let it happen — that they had a bucket to put it in and then they disposed of it. It worked! She allowed her anger and pain to surface and as she cried and yelled, I could feel the tension leave her little body. Later, she told me that she "felt much better now that the tension has gone".

From that point her sessions sometimes developed into 'letting go sessions' quiet and insightful ones, where she talked about her life and how she really felt. She began to use the four emotions in a variety of ways and her emotional growth was staggering. She spoke her truth and about how she feels, accepting responsibility for her feelings and willingly talking about what was happening to her.

Her little sister was totally different, and of course this was inevitable because her start in life was different. She had little parental contact from six weeks on, whereas her older sister had spent two years in the family home.

By the age of five, she had worked out that it was safer for her to be pliable and good and to not speak out. She had learnt to hide 'behind her face'. Her manners were impeccable, and she easily changed from one situation to another, because she had no loyalty or attachment to any one person. In fact, she was later diagnosed with an attachment disorder.

I had been working with her for a while before I realised what she had accomplished for herself and just how deep her fear of abandonment really was. I pointed out to her once how she hid 'behind her face' and that this 'face' showed disdain and seeming insolence. As I worked with her, I often questioned her about this 'face', until, one day, I followed my intuition and offered her a hug. What followed really blew me away! As this little girl screamed and cried, I realised just how deep this fear was and how cleverly she had hidden it from the world. She didn't want anything to do with the angels, she just wanted to deal with it herself. She had become very watchful and aware in her little world and watched her sister, often copying what she had done – a little 'monkey see, monkey do'.

I then began to work with her on activities that focused on 'who am I and what do I have?' I used her as the focus of each activity, so she could see she was worthwhile and real.

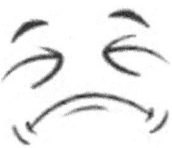

Slowly, she began to talk to me about how she really felt and, if I challenged her at times, she would admit that she was covering up and tell me the truth. I was always very aware how fragile this child's emotional intelligence was and that made me feel very humble. As such, I was very careful of the steps I took as I couldn't afford to let her down.

Helping a child find their place in the world is the greatest privilege a parent has. These souls, who live in little bodies, deserve love and security in order to grow. When a parent or carer can work through their own issues, begin to make changes and let go of toxic patterns of behaviour, their children benefit, even before the parent or carer begins to work with the child. As the process for the child begins, so does the parent/carer's growth continue, as the lessons experienced often challenge them as well.

ENCOURAGEMENT

Acknowledge a child's efforts to help and always thank them. When you make a mistake, if you are able, say "sorry". If a child receives an apology from a parent/carer they learn that it's okay to make mistakes. I watch my son do this with his little boy and my heart sings because my son used to refer to the work I do as, "Mum's hippy stuff". It backs up what I say about when a parent makes changes in their own life, the ripples are never ending.

When you do offer encouragement, make the comment about the child's efforts and intentions rather than the quality of what is produced – "Haven't you done well! Maybe next time we could try it this way."

Physical contact like hugs, gentle ruffling of the hair, or a back rub, can also be encouraging and reassuring. My grandson loves to sit on me as we watch television together, giving him, and me, that physical touch we all need so much.

Share your life with your child. Children need to be included in almost all aspects of a family life and events, such as visiting people in hospital. It's important to talk honestly about illnesses and death without making it too heavy – we do all have to die one day and this is the cycle in which we live.

When a child is included in family life it produces less stress and negates the feeling of being left out. It also introduces children to the realities of life, things that we as parents shy away from that happen every day, such as death and sorrow.

Plan together and try to include children in family decisions. When we moved to a new house, my granddaughter, who was around eight years old at the time, was very stressed until I took her and her sister to see our 'new' house and suggested they choose their own room, thus defusing the stress she felt. Sharing these activities also helped them to look forward to the future.

If you are moving, explain the reason for the move and give them a chance to discuss their feelings and ideas. Sometimes it helps to periodically return to the old area and home after you have moved.

When a new baby arrives, carefully consider which room the baby will sleep in. Perhaps moving an older child from its bedroom could cause resentment and make them feel left out. Talk about the practicalities of a 'new' room – it may be bigger; it can be painted and decorated the way they want. However, it's also important to listen to your child and hear what they have to say about this, as it will save problems later – maybe they don't care if the room is bigger, would rather keep their own room and have the baby sleep in the big room. It's normal for children to become rather possessive over their things and it's important to acknowledge this.

Listening to the child and really hearing what the child has to say, in both words and actions, gives them a sense of security and that they are being heard, reinforcing their emotional security. Children may find it hard to express feelings of fear and confusion, yet they must get these feelings out and know that someone really hears them. Even if you know there is no danger, listen to your child and honour their feelings before offering any other comment.

Bottling up feelings and thoughts can do damage because it prevents the child from growing in awareness and understanding life. Helping a child face up to realities and express their feelings, usually results in greater confidence and the strength to handle life's problems.

Play, drawing, stories, dance, block building, fibre work, can all be used with children to help them explain their feelings. There are some beautiful packages that can add to the tools a parent or carer uses, and these can be bought from any bookstore.

Talking with children and telling them stories about their past, when they ask you to, can sometimes be difficult but it is necessary to answer honestly and limit it to what he can take in. They may not understand the first time you tell them something from the past, so you may need to retell the story a number of times before they understand, before moving on to the next bit.

As a grandparent and carer, I have always tried to answer questions as honestly as I was able and to share the truth where it was appropriate, but only as much as the child was ready to hear. Too much detail, especially about hard topics, such as drugs and violence, can be discussed at a level they are able to understand

When the child grows older and the questions become deeper, my answers have also become more in depth, as the child begins to realise there are more parts to the story.

As a parent or carer, you hopefully know your own child and will learn to gauge the level of detail to include in the answers you give.

I have always believed that one must be truthful and honest with a child. Otherwise how do they ever live to learn their own truth.

> "When I approach a child, he inspires in me two sentiments — tenderness for what he is and respect for what he may become."

— LOUIS PASTEUR

CHAPTER 8
How to Show a Child They are Truly Loved

My deepest belief is that **all** children deserve to be loved, unconditionally. Knowing they are loved, will give a child a real sense of security, space and courage to grow. A child will have confidence knowing that they are okay and that there are people who will love, support, nurture and protect them. Above all, the child will know just how truly special they are.

Knowing they are loved, gives the child confidence in themselves, in the world around them, and helps support their developing nature.

In today's society, family groups come in many different forms. Regardless of the structure of the child's family group, to be loved and cared for by loving nurturing people, is as necessary to the child as breathing.

What makes the child feel loved can differ greatly in our society, where the influence of nurture versus nature is often debated. Regardless, I believe a child who has unconditional love for even only one person, will be happy within themselves and face the world every day with courage.

I would like to offer examples of how a parent/carer in everyday life can show a child they are loved, thus helping them develop loving and caring habits.

Be fully present – with all children, from infants, through to teens, watch them as they talk and move, be very aware of where they are and what they are doing and saying. Body language can tell a parent such a lot when words do not.

Agree with them when you are able. It's also okay to disagree with them if necessary, but do so in a way that the child does not feel put down.

Let them pull out the pots and pans and give them a wooden spoon to bang on them. They can have fun hearing the different sounds, and also get rid of any pent-up emotions they might have.

Play with water as often as you can. Provide all sorts of objects that will carry water. Colour the water with food dye in the sink and let them play while standing on a short stool. Buy cheap water balloons and play outside with them. Throw the water balloons at the fence or a wall.

Understand how brief these few years of childhood are and encourage as many childhood experiences as you can as you will never get these years back. Let your own inner child out and have fun too. Being silly often helps a parent release energy without having to work at it.

Watch favourite cartoons together, snuggled up in a chair. My family love Tom and Jerry and often feel sorry for poor Tom!

Share books every day with your children. Dramatise with your voice while reading and make it fun. Children love the feeling of closeness this story telling gives and it's a wonderful foundation for them when they start learning to read themselves. Kids are non-judgemental when storytelling is happening, so use silly voices and have fun together. Let the child choose the story, and, even if you have to read the same book every night, it's the act of sharing and doing something together that's important.

Share your favourite childhood books with them and teach them how to care for books. Take them to the library and let them choose their own books. It doesn't matter if you don't like the chosen books, it's giving your child a choice that matters. We have also attended story time at various libraries, and this has always been a fun activity to do together.

Honour your child for their great attributes and don't be afraid to tell them how wonderful they are. They won't become vain and the teenage years will be a little easier if they have this self-belief that they're okay just as they are. I always told my youngest son how beautiful he was, especially in those teen years when he was so much taller than his friends.

Reward your child's positive behaviour –the kindness of an older sibling to a younger one.

Find something every day that you like about your child and tell them the things you like and admire. It can be a little hard in those times when they're acting out or you're feeling wronged, so you need to remind yourself that this too will pass, and your loving child will return.

There have been many occasions when I have seen my son apologise after something has been said in anger and the reason for it – "I'm sorry I yelled, it just really annoyed me."

Find the positives in their world and encourage them to find them too: with their friends, their work, the games they play, and the stories they tell.

Make up pleasurable times together – build with boxes and tins, cut and paste.

Never forget just how little and vulnerable they are – you are the adult, the one with experience and this little soul is truly in your care.

Laugh out loud with them, giggle and snigger. Tell them funny stories using their names.

Sing songs – make up silly songs and sing loudly and softly. It doesn't matter if it doesn't make sense. Your child will love it because you're doing it with them.

Feed ducks and swans together. If you have hens, teach them to feed them and gather the eggs.

Be firm when you need to and don't be afraid to say no. This teaches children respect for themselves and for you.

This is sometimes every parent/carer's nightmare as we don't always want to be the 'bad guy'. However, for a child to learn what's right and wrong, we need to be able to stay true to ourselves, be strong enough to wear the fallout and stand firm. As the child grows and learns the meaning of 'no' and that it means no, you will find it easier to be together. This is very much an individual choice for parents/carers and one that you need to think about carefully. If you have a partner, you also have to present a united front and stick together, as children love to divide and conquer.

Help them to understand their feelings – what they are and how to let them go when needed.

Talk about how you feel – not in a deep and meaningful way, just lightly so the child will understand what is happening for you is okay to happen for him.

Learn about and accept your own inner child – allowing them to come out and play too.

Hug many trees – fit your arms around trees together.

Practise deep breathing in games and often.

Build sandcastles and let your child play in the mud and remember, it does wash off with water.

In one of my schools I had a family of three boys whose mother was a meticulous housekeeper and her boys were not allowed to do many things. One day I introduced them to wet clay and one of the little boys spent ten minutes just looking at the clay and wringing his hands together. Finally, he put his hands into the clay very gingerly but I don't think he enjoyed the experience. Interestingly his little brother loved it and got right into the fun of the activity.

When you make a mistake, tell your child you're sorry. If an adult can admit they're wrong and say sorry to a child, the child will learn how to adapt it for themselves. We are only human and sometimes we make mistakes. We do things without thinking and if we can admit we are wrong then the child will know that mum and dad are not perfect, and that it's okay to make mistakes.

Cook together – biscuits that are rolled and cut out, easy cakes and sausage rolls, let them even have a go at putting the ingredients in by themselves.

I knew a lass who had two little boys and found rearing them a great challenge as her husband did not believe in discipline of any sort. One day, when I visited, she had the two boys at the bench, aprons on, and they were making cakes. She had put out the ingredients and let them go, as she watched. I must admit I squirmed as I watched the eggs go in, shell and all, however I knew from my own experiences with the girls, if you persevered, accepted the mistakes and helped them gain good results, in the long run it all paid off. Both of my girls can cook full meals as well as cakes and are very good at having a go at something new.

Walk at your child's pace. One of the very first lessons I remember with children is they can be so incredibly slow, so it's important to slow down yourself and measure your pace to theirs. Go to the park and play on the equipment. Run fast and slow with them. Have races with them and don't always let them win.

Thank them for coming to visit and when they do something to help you.

Ask their opinions about things, such as the colour they'd like their room painted. They have to sleep there, not you.

Listen to them – make eye contact and really hear what they are trying to verbalise.

Set boundaries for their behaviour and stick to them. Talk to them about boundaries and what they are and why we have them, in simple terms, a child is able to understand.

Support your partner when they make a decision, even if you don't agree with it, this shows children they cannot divide their parents for their own ends. Children learn very quickly who the 'softie' is and they tend to go to that person when a decision needs to be made. Talk with your partner when alone and work out between you what the expectations are.

Show them photo albums of their past, their parents and their friends. Keep the photo albums out so they can look when they want to. This may be an issue now with digital cameras, but there needs to be photos available and on display so children know they are worthy.

Build ships and cars, from saved cardboard boxes and cardboard rolls, any other recyclable things you find around the house, or pick up craft items from a two dollar shop.

Build cubby houses together, using the table and chairs, blankets and sheets. When the girls first came to me, Dakota would build a cubby house every day. We often ate our lunch under the kitchen table, which we covered with a sheet, creating a cubby house.

Eat your lunch somewhere, apart from home, perhaps outside under a tree together, or go for a picnic and let your child choose the place.

Share your thoughts and dreams and talk to your child about what they mean to you. Do you have happy dreams or scary ones? When your child tells you about their dreams, listen without judging.

Be crazy – Do crazy things together, as long as you are safe. Perhaps go to the park in your pyjamas!

Talk to your God, depending on your beliefs and the deity you pray to. It doesn't need to be heavy stuff, just something to give your child a sense of spirituality and another dimension for their ideas.

Introduce the concept of angels, or something that can help your child when they are lonely or scared.

Talk quietly and don't yell at your child. I hear you say, "if only I could!" Children can challenge us at times, push us to our limits so we do end up yelling. However, if and when you are able, keep the level of your voice even.

Paint their bodies, in bathers, and yours too, with body paint, then wash it off with the hose.

Have an easel ready to paint on. You can buy cheap ones, together with plastic smocks, at any department store. Otherwise, use the back of a cupboard, the fence, an outdoor wall, to put up large pieces of paper for painting and finger paint.

Use positive language always and **no put downs**, ever. Always tell your child that they are beautiful, unique, special and gorgeous.

When your child does something you don't like, tell them what you don't like – don't label them.

Thank them for good behaviour when you are out. I often used to thank my grandson because he was always beautifully behaved when I took him out. Only twice in four years did he have a meltdown. I took him into the local shopping centre, through a different door, and he couldn't work out where we were, so he yelled at me. When he had cooled down, I told him that this was not how he usually behaved and was he able to find himself in this loud angry person? It turns out he was more scared than angry and this was the only way he knew how to deal with it.

Not all children react like this. Some may behave perfectly in front of other people, with parents experiencing the worst of their child's behaviour when they get home. This can be hard on parents and sometimes children can be nasty. Don't beat yourself up if this happens to you – it's okay to be firm when your child is screaming verbally or physically.

Start teaching them when they are young – take them out and teach them what behaviour you expect, and just remember, it is not always going to be perfect.

Always be genuine in your praise – children very quickly pick up on insincerity.

Every day tell them how much you love them and randomly steal kisses.

Plant flowers and vegetables together and watch them grow. Enjoy, together, the wonderful taste of freshly picked peas.

As you hang the clothes on the line, allow your child to pass you the clothes and the pegs, talking to them as you do this, about the clothes and the warmth of the sun.

Spend quiet time together, listening to music, or simply to the quietness.

Paint the house with water and large brushes.

Tickle each other.

Hang their photos on the wall, all around as each stage changes.

Hang their paintings and drawings where they can be seen. Later save them to use as wrapping paper.

Hug your children often, rolling on the floor together.

Let them ride on your back up the hallway, if you're able.

Let them walk on your feet, as you walk forward, holding them closely to your body.

Play in the rain.

Jump in puddles. This was something I had the greatest pleasure teaching my two granddaughters – Puddles are for jumping in, and we can get clean afterwards. I did the same with swishing through autumn leaves as we shuffled through, not caring what anyone else thought.

Paint white peaked caps and decorate them with glitter and pretty stones. Today there are plenty of two dollar stores around so when you see craft items, buy them, and store them so you have a supply when called upon.

Allow the child to help you as you are working outside in the garden, or in the house. My son was making a new path recently and he had a small pair of gloves and earmuffs for his young son. He told him what he wanted him to do, as he had planned small tasks for him to do, and, as he worked alongside his dad, his dad told him what a great job he was doing.

Engage your child in your interests which don't have to be artistic. Regardless of your hobbies, there are plenty of ways to involve your child so you can spend quality time together. My son shares his interest in Lego with his little boy and they work together. Their mother also involves the children in her garden plans, talks with them about what they can do and gives them space to grow their own plants.

There are so many other ways to show your child they are loved by the people they love back. Use your creative mind to find these ways, allow yourself to let go of adult inhibitions and enjoy sharing fun times with your children.

Making a child feel loved can also give you a tremendous sense of accomplishment and peace. Most of us have children because we want them, so we always want to give them the best of our lives together.

From my many years as a schoolteacher, I rejoiced to see children who knew they were dearly loved — they were confident and able to share themselves with others. Those who were quiet and came across as comfortable and secure, were the children who had support at home.

Another way to show your child they are truly loved and important to you is to become involved at school, if you're able. When parents came to school for canteen duty, or as reading and classroom helpers, their children would look so pleased and happy they were there.

> "Children are one third of our population and all of our future."
>
> — SELECT PANEL FOR THE PROMOTION OF CHILD HEALTH, 1981

CHAPTER 9
Abuse

Sadly, in today's world many people are victims of daily abuse, in one form or another. Sometimes they're not even aware it's happening, or the damage that can result from it. Women, in particular, are vulnerable, with some tragically losing their lives when the abuse becomes out of control.

Some people in ordinary, everyday relationships suffer abuse in various forms and are not aware the abuse is really happening and the danger around them. Often, their abuser doesn't realise what they're doing is wrong and other people can't actually see what's happening in the relationship. Abuse can be very insidious.

For me, this word 'abuse' makes me feel hurt and unsafe – I see an abuser as someone who is out of control.

I found it very hard to write this chapter as it has brought up my own personal experience of violent events in my own life. I am not talking exclusively about violent abuse, just the everyday happenings that people take for granted as being part of daily life.

For me, abuse is when someone is hurt in some way by someone else. It can be physical, mental, sexual or emotional, it can also be very serious and overt or subtle. Regardless of the way a person experiences abuse, there is always someone who ends up hurting. The effects of abuse can be terribly destructive as our cells hold all these traumatic memories, until we uncover them and deal with the stored energy.

Sadly, many of our children are also victims of abuse. Parents would be horrified if they were accused of abusing their children, yet sometimes this happens in subtle ways. Some parents may justify their behaviour by arguing, "this is the way I was brought up and if it was good enough for me, it's good enough for my kids." However, there's a very fine line between discipline and abuse as there's still pain caused to the child.

I need you to understand here that I am not suggesting parents hurt their children on purpose, and I use the word, 'abuse' for shock value – to ask you to stop and think about what you do in your family and to understand just how deeply a child can be hurt when a parent makes a casual comment not meant to hurt, but does.

Sadly, we all carry some hurt from the past. Things that were never true have lodged themselves inside our psyche and become our 'truth' – a truth that we know is not accurate in our hearts but our memory and our heads tell us otherwise. My brother always called me 'fat' – he introduced me to his older friends as 'fat' and taught his young son to call me 'Aunty Fat'. As a result, I had this internal picture of an obese person and it took many years to throw this image off, as I knew it was not really true.

Children at school can also be put down by a careless teacher. When a child offers their thoughts and the teacher pushes it aside with a dismissive comment, this memory can stick. Similarly, getting a child to read out loud in front of the class when they're not a good reader, can have devastating effects on a child later in life. I sometimes ask my older clients, "What are some of the lies you have heard about you that are really not true?"

This has probably been the hardest chapter for me to write as I have lived with children whose lives have been affected by this abuse. I have taught children and worked with clients who have deep scars from comments made early in their lives, having a detrimental impact on their adult life.

WHAT IS ABUSE?

Abuse can be physical, which includes being beaten, slapped, smacked and kicked. Children witness abuse when they see their parents slap or hit each other.

In the past children were strapped with thin pieces of leather and, in many schools, this was the most frightening thing a child could experience. I remember boys hiding the teacher's strap and paying the price when it was found. I know there were times when teachers would use a thirty centimetre wooden ruler to smack children's knuckles. I was even guilty of using a ruler to smack some children who had let their student teacher down at an important time for her.

Fathers would use their belts to strap a child and my mother used a wooden hearth brush on us. Her regular command to us each night was to, "come inside and bring a stick".

Slaps were a common way of getting a child to do what the adult wanted, and I have seen many people slap their child around the head, or across the face.

We hear in the news about the children who have been sexually assaulted by the very people who were in a position to care for, love them and keep them safe.

Emotional Abuse

Emotional abuse comes in many forms and these are just some examples:

Being screamed at.

Being laughed at.

Being told that feelings are not okay – that it's wrong to be angry.

Name calling.

Sarcasm and ridicule.

A parent not being a role model for their child.

A child having to 'parent' a parent.

Not expressing emotion in front of your child.

Not giving your child your time or attention.

Not giving your child direction, limits or boundaries.

Threatening your child with abandonment.

Ignoring your child by not communicating with them.

Emotional abuse is sometimes very hard to be aware of as it's often so easy to make a comment without really thinking about what it will mean to the child. Children feel terrible if they're told their feelings are wrong — "you're stupid to feel like that, you're wrong to be so angry". Parents will sometimes scream at children in anger and despair, threatening them with violence or abandonment, not really understanding that with these comments, they're actually abandoning their child.

Children are sometimes labelled with sarcastic names that can hurt them — my father-in-law named my husband and me, 'Initiative' and 'Sieve Head,' because we didn't do things his way.

Some children also suffer abuse at the hands of other family members, not just the parents. Demeaning comments from relatives can hurt the child and leave deep scars.

I heard a grandmother call her four-year-old granddaughter 'that thing,' one day, in the child's presence and observed the pain on the child's face.

Abuse can also occur when a parent leans heavily on a child, or lets the child make decisions and perhaps run the household. The parent allows their own emotions to become overwhelmed and, therefore, the child ends up parenting the parent. How many times have you heard someone say about their young son, "now he's the man of the house," when he should be allowed to be himself and a child? Although many single mums try very hard to make sure their boys aren't given this responsibility, for some it does continue to happen.

There are also young children in our world today who have to become the carers of their parent or sibling, and this is truly a sad situation for a child.

Some parents do not give their children time, attention, directions, limits and boundaries. When this happens, the child does not develop a good sense of self and may find themselves unable to make their own decisions.

Sexual Abuse

Sexual abuse occurs in a variety of ways and is often accompanied by a deep sense of guilt when a child is told by an adult, "it's our secret and you will not tell anyone".

Abuse can include:

> *Overt touching, contact by rubbing.*
>
> *Exhibitionism; lack of privacy.*
>
> *Voyeurism.*
>
> *Telling children inappropriate, 'dirty' jokes.*
>
> *Referring to a child as a 'surrogate spouse' – innuendos.*
>
> *Grilling a teenager on their sexual behaviour.*

Abuse can happen when the adult rubs the child inappropriately, or bathes the child when it's not necessary. Adults showing themselves in various stages of undressing to the child, or not respecting the child's privacy when they are in the bathroom, toilet or their bedroom, may constitute abuse.

In many families, some fathers have found themselves worrying about their relationships with their daughters because of the many stories in the media about sexual predators. It's a sad indictment on our society that a father can't hug his daughter, regardless of age, the same loving way they are able to hug their sons, for fear they'll be accused of doing so for sexual gratification.

It is also important to give children accurate information regarding sex and not dismiss or joke about the questions they ask about their sexual development – "Hey mum, what's a wet dream?" It's natural for a child to be curious and we need to treat their questions with the greatest respect.

Social Abuse

Restrictions from interaction with peers.

Restrictions on bringing peers home.

Made to wear funny and strange clothes.

Not being taught appropriate manners.

Abuse from peers – "You're fat! You smell!"

Sexism and racism.

Parents can cause this when they put restrictions on children in ways that are not really fair to the child: not allowing a child to interact with their peers; not being able to invite friends home; embarrassing the child in front of their friends; not teaching the child appropriate manners.

Parents can also let their child down innocently when they dress them differently, in garish, outdated clothes, so the child's peers call them names and isolate them.

Other children will also pick up on poor personal hygiene so teaching your child good habits in this area and making sure they go to school bathed and well-presented is important. Similarly, it's important to be aware of the stigma for children if they go to school with head lice. My youngest son, in his first year at school, was not allowed to stand near the teacher because he had head lice, even though I had him at home and his hair was clean. All of this is not meant as abuse, however for the child, it can be shaming and embarrassing.

Intellectual Abuse

This occurs when a child's intellect is questioned and undermined. This may occur when:

> *Parents are unavailable to help with schoolwork and provide answers to questions.*
>
> *Parents don't teach problem solving and assist with task completions.*
>
> *Parents have angry outbursts when the child does not or cannot learn.*
>
> *Verbal put downs when the child's work is presented.*
>
> *A child's values, opinions and ideas are discounted and shamed.*
>
> *Addicted parents who allow the child to witness them using their drug of dependence.*

'Intellectual abuse' is a hard concept to pinpoint and many parents may feel offended that I have included this under the broader heading of abuse. This is because when we try to help our children with their school work, we believe we're doing them a great service, and often we are. Many children learn more at home than they do at school.

Don't get me wrong. I fully support parents' help, but there are some occasions where a parent may use the wrong language when trying to help their child. For example, they may get angry when the child hasn't learnt their spelling for the week, or not completed set work.

Some parents don't have the skills themselves to provide answers and help with homework tasks, or they may be exhausted after a day's work. If this is the case, explain the situation to your child. So often it's **how** you say things to your child, rather than **what** is being said.

Fortunately, for today's parents Mr. Google is there to help. I have found this to be such a fantastic tool for information – children can use it easily, as can we oldies. I find it useful when I come across a word, I am not sure of the meaning, of or while writing this book, the right word for the sentence.

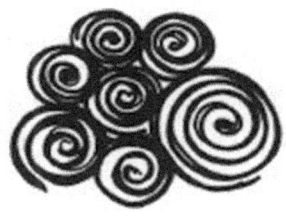

Spiritual Abuse

Convincing a child it's not okay to be human and make mistakes.

Unrealistic rules, or no rules.

Abusive caretakers.

Threats – "You won't go to heaven."

Role models who hold rigid religious beliefs.

Spiritual abuse may happen in a home where religion is the focal point of the parents' lives, often demanding the child follow their rules, even when they are unrealistic. Some rules imply that it's not okay to be human and make mistakes – if the child does not comply, they may be told they will not go to heaven. In some religious sects, a child who leaves the fold is cut right off and shunned. This can sometimes fill a child with great fear and a sense of abandonment.

In our world, we see many instances where religious fervour is being used as a form of spiritual abuse, so it's important to be aware of this when introducing children to religion. For far too long there has been abuse, spiritual and sexual in particular, where children have suffered terrible and lasting consequences. As parents, we must be very aware of how we deal with issues of spirituality in the home. We must also not beat ourselves up when we have an error of judgement. If the very basis of our family life is love, and we maintain connections within the family group, our children will forgive our errors and always love us.

I must add here that when our children go through their teens, we will be faced with challenges we'd rather not deal with. Parents and carers, during these years, are often tried to their limit as they deal with the inevitable struggles that occur as our children emerge as young adults. However, it's my experience, and that of many other parents, that these years will pass and the values we instilled in our teens, when they were little, do play a part and are not totally lost. These children do survive and hopefully come out the other end of this experience with greater maturity. As their carers, we are also given the opportunity to strengthen our relationships and our emotional connections with them.

Once again I would like to borrow from the work of life coach and therapist, Nicholas de Castella, who explains, in his article,

'At War With Children,' different forms of parental anger and how children react to it:

When a parent is angry with a child or feels that they at war with them, the adult attacks by using:

Personal criticism: "You look like a tart in that outfit!"

Accusations: You broke the picture, didn't you?"

Sarcasm: "Of course! You know it all!"

Blaming: "It's your fault your sister is crying!"

Generalising: "You're just like your mother/father!"

Dismissive comments and gestures:
"P... off! Let the professional do it!"

Mean comments and put downs: "What a stupid idea!"

Comparisons: "Why can't you be more like your sisters?"

Sharp and abrupt commands: "Get over here now!"

Cold shouldering and not talking.

Running late to drop them off or pick them up.

Refusing to help: "Do it yourself!"

The tone of voice used in these messages also gives the child a fair warning of what the adult is saying and when accompanied by aggressive, angry body language, the child **knows** they are under 'attack' and will often go into defensive mode by:

- Running away from the situation and maybe hiding.
- Being quiet and making themselves 'small' so they are less likely to be noticed.
- Trying to please.
- Apologising excessively.
- Withdrawing from the situation.
- Making excuses for their behaviour.
- Rebelling against the adult.
- Being insolent.
- Denying the behaviour.
- Displaying either extremely good or bad manners.
- Crying easily.

It's important to never underestimate a child's feelings, or their understanding of a situation.

BLAME AND SHAME

Although I discussed the topics of blame and shame in Chapter 7, I believe it's important to also include it when discussing abuse. Blaming and shaming are often forms of abuse and need to be highlighted as such.

Just to reiterate; shame is an 'e–motion', in other words, energy in motion. It can be healthy or unhealthy.

Healthy shame is the feeling we get when we make an honest mistake and the purpose of this type of shame is to remind us of our essential humanity – that, as humans, we can, and do make mistakes.

Sometimes, there is a mismatch between what we need as children, and what our parents/carers are able to provide. This, in part, results from the pressure people feel to be a good parent, spouse, provider – all the roles adults are expected to fulfil when they have children. In trying to fulfil these societal expectations, at times, parents may become either, 'less than human' – resulting in rage, incest, assault – or 'more than human' – becoming over-achieving, self-righteous and critical.

These expectations may lead parents to not be present when the child needs their care. The child may then feel abandoned as they're too young to either understand what's happening, or to resolve these issues on their own.

I'd like to repeat and highlight some common areas of life where we are often shamed and are often verbally abused because of it.

Our bodies: too thin; too fat; too tall, too short, wrong shaped nose wrong shaped ears, haircuts, skin colour.

Our feelings: too emotional, a sook, not emotional enough, too dramatic, too complex, too moody, a 'drama queen'.

Our intellect: too "dumb", too "stupid", too intellectual, a 'nerd'.

Our sexuality: not dressing appropriately, too 'slutty', too 'prudish', blamed for being gay, straight, bisexual, virgin. Hearing statements like: "Can't you cover up and look decent!"; "If you masturbate, you'll go blind"; "Don't dress like that. You look like a tart."

As I have said earlier in the book, it's important to acknowledge our own shame and begin to deal with it. Acknowledging it and seeing it as we experienced it in the past helps bring it out of the darkness and into the light. It exposes it and this helps let shame go so we can be free.

Simple words can create a life-long impact. For example, for me being called "stupid" by my mother had a huge shaming effect on me that took me a long time to work through.

Research shows that a healthy internal environment is essential if mental health and disease are going to be reversed – that only happens if one is able to understand how we can take control of our lives.

It is not what happens to you that matters – it is how you deal with it that counts!

Many times during my boys' teenage years, I purposely used that phrase and found that they could relate it to their own lives and understand its meaning.

My oldest son was a surfer. He also suffered dark periods in his life, so I asked him one day, "What do you do when the wave pushes you under the water? Do you stay there and drown, or do you fight your way to the top and start again?"

I also told the girls that they could not use what happened in their early years as an excuse to grow – perhaps a reason why it was challenging, but never an excuse.

From this I learned to deal with blame and shame and, with a small child, I have been able to explain that 'next time you might do it differently' or ask, "What do you think you could do to make it different next time?"

Learn to use constructive criticism when you need to help a child, never destructive. Little minds take in everything you say and, as alternative medicine advocate and author, Deepak Chopra explains – "Everything that happens to us in our lives is stored in our cells, much of which is untrue."

> "If you want your children to be intelligent, read them fairy tales. If you want them to be more intelligent, read them more fairy tales."

ALBERT EINSTEIN

> "I have found the best way to give advice to your children is to find out what they want and then advise them to do it."

— HARRY S. TRUMAN

CHAPTER 10
Heart Truth

For many years now I have been facilitating emotional wellness groups where I have always included an acknowledgement of our hearts. In particular, the importance it plays in our everyday lives and in how we deal with our emotions.

I ask people to put their hands on their hearts, with their eyes closed, and encourage them to allow themselves to feel the love that is in there – the love for others and the love for themselves.

My reason for doing this is to remind people that their heart can be open or closed. Open to the way they love and live their emotional lives and how they react to others, or closed to all emotions, whereby they shut out the world and its meanings.

How many times do we use the word **heart** in our everyday speech?

I don't have the heart to….

My heart aches because…

I was heartened by….

He took heart when….

At a weekend workshop I attended with Nicholas de Castella a few years ago, he instructed the group to point to the roof, then to the floor, then to ourselves. He then asked us where we were pointing and when we looked around the room, everyone pointed to the place where we believe our hearts to be.

So, what is 'heart truth', and how do we encourage children to have it?

I believe when children are born, they come into this world with open hearts. As they grow, they speak from their hearts and they speak their heart's truth.

Sadly, as they grow they learn to close down their truths because often the adults in their lives make it hard for them to stay open and be truly real. Many children don't have enough confidence in their parents to speak their truth because they are often shut down as they try to do so.

I remember often telling my youngest son to "shut up" because I just didn't have the patience for his third lot of questions. However, I rejoice to see him as a father now, listening to what his own children say. I know this is, in part, the influence marriage and family has on him, yet it is still very special to observe this as his mother.

These days, many children don't even have the family together at mealtimes because the television is on, giving the news of the day. This means there's no opportunity for sharing, learning, or just having fun.

One of my friends who believed in talking with her four children and listening to what they had to say, used to ask each one at the table, "What was the best thing that happened to you today?" Each child in that family was listened to and validated and have grown up to be caring and fantastic parents themselves.

Think about what happens at your meal times? Are the people in your household sharing their thoughts, ideas, beliefs and daily happenings? Or, do the children in the family have to sit quietly and have no input?

I understand how tired parents get – tired of the questions and the constant sound of childish voices – but we don't have our children with us for very long and these years pass so quickly.

I also know how tiring it is to have a small child constantly nagging at you to, "play with me, or asking "why, why, why?" However, It's very important to be real here and to ask yourself just how much of this you can do. Ask your family to support you, your friends who know you, and those who will give you an honest answer.

Over the years, my friend June has been my sounding board and when I've had concerns about the girls, she has told me her thoughts, even when she's felt the need to be brutally honest. I have always respected June's opinion as it gives me another perspective.

Being real is having an open heart and mind as well as speaking one's truth from the heart. It's also about being loving and trusting.

My mum told me once that she listened to her mother when she told her what to do, then when she was on her own, she worked things out for herself.

Sadly, for some children, by the time they reach their teenage years, they have mostly closed their hearts because it hasn't been safe to be open and trusting. This means by the time they're adults, blocks are firmly in place.

So, how do we open our hearts and move from out of our minds into our hearts? How do we feel safe to do this?

The first step is to find a safe place where you will not be disturbed. Close your eyes and allow yourself to mentally feel your body. Become aware of the inner sensations you're feeling.

A child can do this just as easily as an adult can and it's good to encourage a child to learn about the feeling state of their body and what this means.

Ask them – "If you're feeling good, where do you feel that in your body?"

Body awareness activities, such as wriggling your toes when asked, placing your hands on different parts of the body, holding your hand over your heart and imagining what it feels like there: "What colour is it, what shape does it have?" These activities can all help a child become aware of their body and how it feels to have stored energy in different parts of it.

I have talked to the girls, and the people I work with, about the love that is in your heart, the love that you can share. I explain that when love comes from the heart, just how good it can be.

From there it's a step to the next level of feeling.

"Where do you feel happy? Where do you feel sad?"

Put your hand on that place and feel the feeling you have. Then visualise the colour of this feeling, the shape and what it looks like. Allow yourself a few moments for this to be felt properly.

Ask your child if they want to talk about this experience, or give them time to draw with crayons, or pencils, on large sheets of paper. Have a sketchpad for them to draw in that can become a continuing record of their work in this area. Make sure you date each drawing, so you can monitor the child's growth.

A child can do this activity as easily as an adult can, and it's good to encourage the child to learn about the feeling state of their body and what it means to them. All this can help a child become aware of their body and how it feels to have stored energy in different parts of it. This is what emotions are – energy within the body.

At the completion of these exercises, ask your child, and yourself – "What is the state of your heart? Is it open to the emotions you feel, express and experience, to the love around you and the feelings that happen every day? Are you open to the peace and serenity love can bring?"

You don't have to be in a relationship with anyone else but yourself to know what love is.

For me and my clients, it's important to know, understand, and accept 'heart truth'.

Ask yourself these questions:

"What is the state of my heart?"

"Is it open to the emotions I acknowledge and experience every day, to the love around me, that is offered to me by the people in my life?"

"Is my heart open to the feelings of peace and serenity love can bring, or, is it closed?"

"Is my heart blocked and shut down as a result of not being able to work with my emotions?"

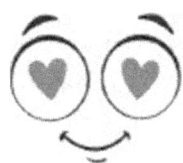

"Does it terrify me by not acknowledging whatever I'm feeling, that's making me anxious or worried?"

"Can I allow myself to open up and learn about myself – what I truly feel, what I need to set myself free?"

*"What is it that I need to do to allow myself
to really feel and set myself free?"*

Imagine, if you can, you are locked away inside a very heavy suit of armour – the type that knights used to wear. Imagine the huge weight of this full armour and helmet, as well as the spear and shield you're carrying. Picture this image and then imagine your heart is tucked away, under all of this armour – not allowed to feel, not allowed to be free.

Ask yourself – *How does this feel? What would it be like to have this armour on for the rest of my life, never being able to be at ease, in your health and in your relationships?*

How does this suit of armour affect my very freedom?

Here I encourage you to close your eyes and look into your heart and to allow any feelings, whether large or small, to be acknowledged. Then, open your heart wide to the changes you wish to make in your life, ask for divine guidance and allow this to happen.

If you feel you are locked away in a suit of armour, allow yourself a space to peel away this suit, piece by piece, until your heart begins to open and let the sunshine in.

Here are some physical ways to help this process:

Find someone who specialises in 'heart counselling' who will work with you. This form of counselling is an integrated approach that uses the healing power of love, compassion and acceptance. It means listening to one's heart and finding one's own inner voice. You can check online to find qualified counsellors in your area, or ask for recommendations from people who are on their own spiritual path.

Buy yourself a piece of rose quartz and place it where you can touch it every day. Rose quartz represents unconditional love, in any form.

Above all, nurture yourself because you need to be able to do this before you can truly help someone else.

According to Nicholas de Castella, there are five steps to being heart centred:

Stop

Stop going anywhere, doing anything. Spend a few moments practising mindfulness. Let yourself settle and be still. Do not try to make anything happen. Just let yourself be still.

Breathe

Spend a few moments practising gentle, relaxed, flowing breathing.

Feel

Note which emotion you are feeling at this moment. Do you feel angry, happy, sad, fearful or blank?

Tune into the actual physical sensation and the location of these feelings.

Allow

Allow the feelings to just be, just as they are, and to change as they may or may not.

Take your focus to your heart

Allow yourself to tune into your heart, in your heart region. Think of someone you love and allow yourself to feel that love. Allow the feeling to grow and welcome it all in as you continue to breathe gently. Gently notice what comes into your awareness. Enjoy this moment as this is all you have.

Be grateful for the love and allow this to enter your consciousness.

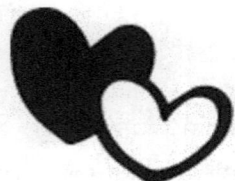

> "While we try to teach our children all about life, our children teach us what life is all about."
>
> ANGELA SCHWINDT

CHAPTER 11
Resilience

What is resilience?
According to the dictionary definition, it's "the capacity to recover quickly from difficulties."

For me resilience is:

Being able to get out of bed in the morning, after a difficult night with a child, and present the best version of myself I can for the day.

Being able to get out of the bed and go to work the next morning, after dealing with desperate phone calls in the middle of the night from my addicted son needing help.

When a child, or husband has been injured, being able to carry on as 'normal,' whilst helping others.

Losing people, you love when they pass over and being able to move through the pain, remaining constant.

Being able to survive a broken marriage or being beaten and physically hurt by someone you love and, for me, countless different scenarios.

Being resilient has meant being able to pick up the pieces after an incident and go on living successfully, knowing the world is a great place.

Throughout my life resilience has always been an important strength I've been able to draw upon. Many times, life dealt me and my family serious blows, which always involved some sort of loss.

Because of this, it has always been imperative that I experience the blows, work though the emotion, then pick myself up and go on. I could not lie down and let life over run me – life was simply too important for me to ever let go and not survive.

As a result, I did develop some serious coping strategies in my life:

I took the word 'try' out of my vocabulary because I believed you either did something or you didn't – there was no 'trying' in this.

I raised my boys and the girls with this mantra – when something happens in life, we have two choices – we can fall down, stay there and become a victim, **or** we 'pull our fingers out' and get back on the job.

"If you fall off your bicycle, what do you do?"

"If your girlfriend dumps you, what do you do?"

And so on, throughout life.

Each time you choose to get back on with your life, you build strong stepping-stones which give you the strength to face life's challenges and support you to overcome difficult changes. In fact, this all means you are becoming **resilient.**

As parents, we begin to help a child develop resilience from a very early age – as they learn to crawl, sit up and walk. We don't let him lie on the floor and stay there. We encourage him to keep working on their efforts.

We then take great pride in the first steps our child takes as they develop. We are rewarded by taking pride in our child, as well as enjoying their delight as they discover these new skills.

This learning continues as a child grows and starts school. However, if you complete your child's homework for them because you want them to pass, you may hinder growth as their teacher won't know they're struggling.

Children need to learn success and failure to become resilient.

Teenage years can be the hardest for many parents. Some teenagers think they're the only people in the world who have problems and they allow themselves to be 'smooshed' into the carpet. Many have unsatisfactory relationships with their parents and some have very sad inner pictures. Yet many of these young people will respond to people who care and take a genuine interest in what they're doing. Being listened to and heard is essential when it comes to helping a teen build resilience, especially if they have not yet developed these skills.

Teenagers need boundaries – as much as they push against them, they need to know just how far they can go before an adult will take over.

Sometimes it seems easier to give in and to let go of the need to survive, ultimately becoming a victim, just waiting for the next blow to fall.

Often, it is so hard to get back up, draw up your defences and get back into the life you lead. However, it's necessary to do this if you want to set an example for your children and family, because each time you do this, you develop your own resilience further.

My oldest son, Luke, is the greatest example of resilience I know.

In his early years, he suffered some very nasty accidents, survived and continued to grow. When he was eleven he had a stupid accident that involved a biro going point first, at speed, into his right eye and puncturing it. Harrowing months passed with the loss of sight in that eye. Luke endured two operations, the making and fitting of a prosthetic half eye and finally having to wear glasses, as his other eye was shortsighted. Finding out he needed glasses was the only time Luke cried. Even though he had worn an eye patch to school for months with no problems, the thought of glasses just overwhelmed him.

Even though everything that happened throughout this journey, which involved many hours of travel to appointments, was painful, sad and frustrating, Luke only asked me once, "Why me?". The rest of the time this young boy carried himself with dignity and great courage.

A teacher told him that he would never play cricket again. How wrong some people can be! Luke played, not only cricket – he played golf, football, basketball, was brilliant at table tennis, rode a bike to and from school for years, later rode a motorbike and surfed. Over the years, he got his motorbike and car licence, learnt to drive a forklift and worked on oil rigs, never once saying, "I can't do it".

Resilience and courage have been Luke's strengths and recently his life was rewarded by a beautiful wife and cherished daughter. I have always been so proud of him as it could have been easier to use his accident as an excuse and give up.

My eldest granddaughter, Dakota, now as an adult, also has great resilience. I have walked beside her through a life that has been far from easy, through many hard lessons that would have brought an adult down. Yet, despite all these challenges, she picks herself up the next day with renewed courage and finds solutions.

She has chosen to become a secondary school teacher, teaching boys in years nine and ten, and she continues to grow.

No, it is not always easy to get up each day and keep going, but there are ways you can support yourself and I offer you some here.

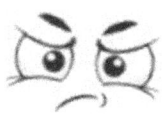

These strategies are based on the work of Doctor Susan Taylor, Director of the Centre for Meditation Science, Pennsylvania, and author of the book *Seven Ways to Build Resilience*. I have added extra details here with her approval.

This practice is known as 'Five Senses Meditation'.

Remain calm

Be consciously aware and live in the moment. Sometimes this is easier said than done when you're in a stressful situation. However, when you can take your mind out of the experience, or after it's over, become very conscious of what's happening right now.

Breathe

Take a deep breath and let it out s-l-o-w-l-y. Take another deep breath, then another, noting what is happening in your body as you do this. Let this breath go and breathe naturally, but keep your awareness within yourself. Become aware of what you can see and see past it, if it hurts.

Listen

Close your eyes and listen. What can you hear?

Feel

What is touching you and is around you? Perhaps it's the wind, sun, stillness or clothing. Use your body as it gives you feedback. What's happening now? What am I feeling? Give it a name, even if it's only a whisper. Where in my body am I feeling it? Welcome the feeling in and surround it with your love.

Smell

What can you smell?

Taste

What is the taste in your mouth?

As you engage in this form of meditation, it becomes easier to pull your awareness back to the present and keep your consciousness in the **now**.

Embrace change

Change can be very scary, as well as exciting, as it's usually something new. As you examine the change, allow yourself to let go of past experiences and memories. Open your heart to let this new experience happen.

Nourish yourself

Make sure you are safe, warm and nurtured. If not, take steps to make this happen.

Build positive social relationships

Let go of toxic people in your life and people who bring negativity into your life. Life is a journey where you meet many people, both negative and positive, all of whom have a role to play in our lives. When people are dark and down there is no place for them in your life. Find new friends and develop sound and happy relationships with positive people.

Look for positive role models and place pictures of them somewhere you can see them every day, such as on the fridge door.

For several years now, I have kept a photo on my fridge of one of my favourite Australian Rules footballers, Tom Hafey. Tom was a footballer and a coach and when he retired from playing, he kept himself as fit as he could. He ran every day, up until his death in his eighties. Having a picture of him on my fridge reminded me I needed to walk or run every day.

Find the purpose in your life

My purpose was always about children and their welfare. When I retired, this purpose widened to include helping those less fortunate than me. I support marginalised women overseas, especially in Nepal, by providing them with sanitary kits. I have also gone to Nepal to visit these women, helping them to sew their own pads. During the recent pandemic lockdowns, I have sewed every day, even if it's only been an hour, making shields, pads and masks. This has helped me to survive this period as each night I can go to bed knowing I've done something I think is worthwhile for the day. I ended up making one hundred kits for one hundred Nepalese girls.

Practise your skills

Acknowledge what it is that you can do and spend time doing it. Open your heart and allow yourself to acknowledge the skills you have. Honour those skills by practising and improving them, perhaps even sharing them with others. I can sew, so I make things for others. I can write, so I have added this chapter to my book.

TEN TIPS FOR BUILDING RESILIENCE IN TEENAGERS

1. Meet with other people, even parents, and ask them questions about how they build resilience in themselves. Listen to their answers and don't be afraid to express your own opinion.
2. When something does happen in your life that 'knocks you off your perch' be kind to yourself and allow yourself to feel what is happening for you without criticism.
3. Make a 'safe' place where you are hassle free and can be alone, such as your bedroom, or you can allow your family/friends in when appropriate.
4. Stay within your normal routines – ones that make you feel good and safe, such as going to school, if school is safe for you. Spend time with friends.
5. Take care of yourself – physically, mentally and spiritually. Get enough sleep to help you through the day.
6. Control your actions – even if you have to move slowly to take control of what you do, such as getting ready to go to school.
7. Allow yourself to express what you feel – perhaps not always talking, but using a journal or doing something creative.
8. Help someone else by volunteering. Help around the house, or help friends with their homework.
9. Put things into perspective – Use your past experiences to help you put the right perspective on what's happening in your life. Learn some relaxation techniques, such as tai chi, meditation or yoga.
10. Turn it off – Even though you want to know about daily life, don't constantly watch and read the news. Keep up with the news with one report daily and turn off the rest.

I used this technique during the recent COVID outbreak in Victoria. Although I wanted to know the main details, I didn't want to hear all the commentary and stories repeated, which can be highly stressful, so I chose to watch only one news program a day.

Take small steps, one at a time, so you know you are accomplishing something. Start small and add to it as you begin to feel more comfortable. Ask for help if needed. Take one idea you can work with and follow through – for example: when I get out of bed, I'll have a shower, get dressed and go for breakfast.

Develop your own 'box of tricks' or a 'toolbox' such as yoga, tai chi, meditation, music, drawing, anything that helps you relax.

Be flexible – If what you're doing is not working for you, change it.

Always be aware of your words – For example, change, "I can't ride my bike up the hill as well as dad does" to "look how far up the hill I rode". Be conscious of always using positive language.

Accept support – It's okay to ask for it when you need it and it's okay to provide support for someone else. When you feel you can't go on, ask some you trust for help – they will feel good being able to help too.

Develop gratitude – Daily gratitude helps us to become more resilient. My day begins with my gratitude statements – "I'm grateful I woke up today; for this house I live in; that the sun is shining." It sets the tone of the day and I can then get up and feel ready for whatever will come.

Remind yourself of past times you have successfully come through negative times, how you did it and how you can

adapt those skills for now. I remember that I closed my eyes, concentrated on slowing my breathing, mentally letting go of the tension in my body.

GRATITUDE

For me gratitude is an emotion that makes me thankful, happier and more in tune with the world.

According to the dictionary definition: "gratitude is a feeling of appreciation felt by someone, or a similar positive response shown by the recipient, of kindness, gifts, help, favours, and other types of generosity, towards the giver of such gifts".

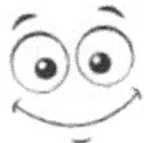

People can easily and consciously cultivate gratitude in their lives and especially in children's lives. Children have so much in today's world so it's important to teach them about gratitude. Without making it heavy, a parent can talk to a child about what there is to be grateful for, such as their families and the fact they're living in a peaceful, safe country.

HELPING CHILDREN CULTIVATE GRATITUDE IN DAILY LIFE

Begin by asking your child the things in their life that bring them happiness? These things can range from simple things, to deep thanks – "I'm thankful I can go back to school."

Make little 'thank you books' with your child and get them to write down the things they are grateful for.

Encourage your child to write in a daily journal, recording the things they are grateful for, both the big and the small.

Ask your child to find three things that have gone well for them this week – Perhaps it's something as simple as getting to ride their bike with their friend.

As adults, we can also do this. Begin a list with all the things you are thankful for, starting with your everyday life and extending as you find other things to add to your list.

Personally, I am grateful that winter is over. I am grateful that I've had the opportunity to travel, something I love, and been able to enjoy the journey – the places I visit and the people I meet. I am so thankful for my gypsy spirit but also feel the deepest gratitude as my plane comes in to land and I know I'm back on Australian soil.

Begin each day with gratitude. At the age of seventy-seven, I am always grateful to wake up.

Smile more often. Practise by smiling at your face in the mirror.

Find inspiring people in the world and read their stories. One of my favourites is a book by cancer survivor, Jess Van Ziel, called *Eye Won*.

Jess's story is a story of great loss, pain and sadness, as well as success and joy. Jess is one of the most positive and resilient people I have ever met and she just brims with life. Her story will show you how a young person can turn their life around from darkness and loss, to one of happiness with gratitude and positivity. Her resilience continues to bring her success and great love.

Acknowledge the beauty of nature. The sea, the sky and all its glory.

Become conscious of how you communicate and what comes out of your mouth.

Look for the positives in everything you do.

When something hard happens, look at it critically and ask yourself, what can I learn from this?

When teaching your children to be grateful, make it simple.

Encourage them to thank mum or dad for a cooked meal. Compliment them when they are positive.

Quietly remind them to be conscious of the words they speak.

Make a gratitude poster using pictures and photos and put it up where your child can see it every day.

I remember in many of the courses I have done, I was asked to make charts listing what I wanted to achieve and have in the future, or what my goals were, an activity I found quite challenging.

Recording what I am grateful for would be a lot easier and the list would be endless!

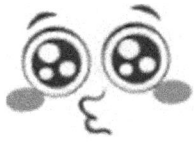

EMPATHY

What is empathy?

According to the dictionary definition: "Empathy is the ability to understand and share the feelings of others."

Empathy is a key element of emotional intelligence — it is the link between us, as humans, as we understand what another person is feeling, just as if we were feeling it ourselves.

Empathy is different to sympathy, which is feeling sorry for someone else, bringing out our own emotions.

Empathy means 'feeling with' the other person, by being able to understand, or relate to, their feelings and reactions. Empathy can also come from sharing similar personal experiences. It's a feeling that can be developed if a person does not already have it.

Helping our children develop empathy lies mainly in our ability to talk with them about other children's experiences and asking them how they would feel if a certain thing happened to them.

Children will need support in this area as it is not something a child will immediately understand — sympathy may be easy for them but empathy may need more explanation. As a child's emotions tend to change so quickly, there may only be fleeting opportunities to share this experience and explain what is meant by empathy.

Teaching your child to be self-aware can help teach them about empathy.

Encourage your child to slow down, stop and breathe deeply.

Find the feeling, acknowledge it and give it a name.

Find a way to release the feeling, by breathing in and blowing it out. Other breathing exercises I have described in earlier chapters, may also help your child achieve this release.

Doing these exercises can help your child to become self-aware of not only their own feelings, but the feelings of their friends.

Meditation is another effective way to learn self-awareness.

You can use short meditation exercises with your child, such as 'The Five Senses Meditation', and bring your child's awareness back to the moment you are in.

Encourage your child to stop, close their eyes and breathe. Ask them what's happening for them at that moment. Get them to 'feel' their hands, feet, fingers, followed by giving their body a really good shake, and letting go.

> "Children are great imitators. So give them something great to imitate."

— ANONYMOUS

CHAPTER 12
Ways Children Learn About Life

The ways in which patterns are set early in a child's life, the way they are reared and the behaviour they witness is how they learn about life.

When parents are understanding and tolerant, children learn to be patient.

When parents are open and supportive and praise their child, a child learns appreciation.

When parents show unconditional love and acceptance, the child learns to love.

When parents encourage their child, the child learns to be brave and to try again.

When parents show approval, the child learns to like and trust themselves, as well as their choices.

When parents share, give freely of their time and their talents with children, the child learns the path to sharing with others.

When parents recognise their child and their efforts in a positive way, the child can begin to set goals.

When parents are honest and live their truth, the child learns to understand what their own truth is.

When parents are fair with their children, set boundaries and support each other's decisions, a child learns about justice and being supportive to others.

When a child lives in an environment of love, friendliness and acceptance, the child learns they are okay, and that the world **is** a great place to live in.

When a child lives in a home that honours **all** of its inhabitants, they learn about self-acceptance.

When a child lives in a home where their efforts are accepted and talked about, the child learns about self-confidence.

When a child lives in a home where they are acknowledged for their inner beauty, a child learns about self-esteem.

In a home where parents criticise each other, their children and other people in their lives, the child learns to condemn and criticise themselves and others.

When parents are hostile and violent, the child learns how to fight and about mistrust.

When parents have a fear of something or somebody, the child learns apprehension – a fear of water, for example, may mean a child is not confident in swimming.

When a child lives in a house where self-pity is encouraged, the whole family becomes victims and feel sorry for themselves.

When a child is ridiculed and put down, they become afraid to show their true feelings and become shy and withdrawn, or, alternatively, aggressive with other children.

When there is jealousy in a house, a child can learn what guilt feels like.

When parents are angry with each other and the world, the child understands rage.

What are the lessons in your world that your children are learning about?

IN CONCLUSION

Originally, my goal in writing this book was to share my many years of experience working with children and the successful strategies I have used to help them understand and deal with their emotions. As I revise this work, I have been writing for several years. I believe now, more than ever, all children need support in learning about their emotions – what they are, how they affect our lives and how to simply deal with them and let them go.

No-one needs to be controlled by their emotional baggage. This baggage can be dealt with and the stifling power of letting it go, and releasing the pain and hurt it causes.

Children have always been my passion. I believe they are the most important people in our lives and I have been blessed over and over by the ones I have reared and worked with.

Each child is unique, each deserves the best we can give them. Each child also needs to learn to understand emotions and how important they are in life.

We only have our children for such a very short time and I believe they are only lent to us. As the poet, Kahlil Gibran wrote:" You are the bows from which your children as living arrows are sent forth."[3]

It is our privilege to rear these children and we should be committed to make the years we have together the very best we can.

Emotional wellness and intelligence go hand in hand – understanding the power of emotions and how they work equals wellness and happiness always.

When I set out to discover why my head ached so intolerably all those years ago, and, coming from a background where all I knew was 'black and white', anger and no anger, it was the start of a fascinating challenge. A challenge that lead me to an understanding that emotional wellness can be at the base of great happiness and also great *dis- ease*.

For me, it was not an easy journey because I fought against many personal, deep seated beliefs and paradigms. It wasn't until I let go of the need to always be in control, no matter what, and discovered that there was an easier and happier way to walk through this world of mine.

It still isn't always easy but I'm happier and freer now and it's all to do with letting go and the need to be right. I understand now that it's easier to be happier when I recognise and honour how I'm feeling.

As I worked with the children at the beginning of my emotional journey, I knew what I was doing could be easily adapted and accepted by the other children I met along the way. That they would learn to acknowledge their emotions, without judgement, accept them and let them go, in a safe environment.

My work with children also gave them the freedom to play with different ways of releasing emotions, to have fun during the experience and feel the benefit after it was all over.

As my granddaughter Summer used to say, after whacking and smacking the bed with the toy baseball bat, "I feel so much better now." I have had clients say, "I feel so much lighter now," and my grandson said, after he had punched out his anger, "I feel all soft now".

Sometimes there can be **huge** parental fear when you embark on this work, which is natural as I'm suggesting you change the way you think and challenging your beliefs.

These are the beliefs that have supported you as a parent, until now, which you probably learned from parents who also didn't know just how important emotional intelligence is. So, all I suggest is that you take each step into this world slowly and carefully, but also with great trust in the process, and in yourself, as you're directing it.

Talk about this with your partner, if you're in a relationship, or to a trusted person if you are not. Above all, trust your instincts. You know your own child and your goal is to benefit them and make life easier.

As you do this, you can only build stronger and better relationships with your children and help them learn to help themselves.

Our society does not always accept people who are emotionally intelligent or aware and there will always be those who laugh, sneer or try to put you down. However, the people most likely to criticise you are often scared of their own truths.

If you can put this criticism aside and embrace the challenge of helping your child become emotionally intelligent, you're giving them, and yourself, the greatest gift imaginable.

To be emotionally intelligent and well, one needs to be humble – to be prepared to look inside themselves and to honestly accept who they really are. If you can do this then you are well on your way to better health and happiness.

By way of recap, these are the emotions you need to understand so you are able to successfully manage them.

Anger is the energy of strength. Anger gives you strength to get things done – puts fire in your belly as you face opposition, and the energy to make changes.

In my world it is bright red and I often wear red scarves to lift the black clothes I sometimes wear.

It is the energy of spring – the way of new growth, pushing through the ground to be seen, the new life that forces its way out of the womb, to face reality. The forces of nature that bring change. Remember, I am not talking about rage here, only the energy that healthy anger creates.

Joy is the energy of happiness and light. Joy accepts that life is good – that great things happen; that success is there for those who choose to accept it; that great love is possible and great achievements will bring glory and gladness.

In my world it is yellow, the energy of summer, where everything shines in the light of the bright sun – where there are only bright skies and life. Joy is an emotion that challenges me to explore, create, love and have fun.

Sadness is the energy of loss, grief and darkness. It is the energy of winter, when the trees lose their leaves and become bare, the days shorten so we feel locked away in the dark. It is cold and some of us can't get warm – old people have to stay inside as they're unable to brave the cold outside, becoming housebound and often sad. We mourn the stark bare trees and the sadness of loss.

I have watched five of my beautiful friends experience this energy during the past year, as each one has lost her partner to death. I have seen grief in all its 'glory' which has highlighted the fact that this is an emotion we all feel in our lives, and to experience it fully we must allow, allow, allow. For me, the emotion of sadness is dark, dark navy blue in colour.

Fear is the energy of losing something valuable – of not knowing what is going to happen next, of how our lives might change as we have no control with being hurt.

It is the energy of autumn, when the leaves fall and the warmth disappears – the seesaw of days with warmth and cold, not knowing just what to expect next. What will happen when/if? How will I deal with it? Can I cope? What will I do? How will it affect my life? What will happen to me?"

For me fear is the colour brown and I feel very low and slow if I ever wear dull brown. It makes me feel like a nameless, unhappy little sparrow who doesn't want to be noticed in the world. I am colourless, so, therefore, I am not important, or included in this world.

Nothingness – I have not felt this often as I am a very emotional person. I cannot shut my feelings down. Even when I lived in China and made a conscious decision to not show my true feelings, I still felt them deeply.

Nothingness means just that – nothing, shut down, meaningless, nowhere, indifference, passive, detachment, lethargy, empty, apathy.

For me, black is the colour of this feeling as I believe this colour is worn to hide behind, to cover all emotional energy.

Interestingly, black can often be a corporate colour, so perhaps this is an environment where the feelings hide?

The list below contains words I'd like you to consider – how you use them, how you understand them and which group you think they belong to. Be aware that some can fit in to more than one category:

grumpy	*alarmed*	*hostile*
regretful	*saddened*	*euphoric*
sobbing	*amused*	*withdrawn*
delighted	*serious*	*upset*
upset	*moody*	*hesitant*
fuming	*passionate*	*offended*
cheery	*carefree*	

Regardless of how you have categorised these words, you have done well as this was an exercise to see if you have learned any differences in your emotional world.

There are no rights or wrongs, whatever you did was perfect for you at this moment in time.

Lastly, I would like you to sit there and be mindful of where you are right now, in the present, in the **now.**

Close your eyes, become aware of your breathing and allow yourself to sit in this state of awareness.

Now ask yourself:
What's happening in my body right now?
What is the feeling?
Where is it?
How does it make me feel?
Thank you, self.

Open your eyes and look around, feeling gratitude for who you are and what you have – that you have had the courage and interest to read something that may help you to change your life and the life of your child.

So, thank you for reading and good luck in sharing your own emotional awareness with yourself and your family.

And remember, emotional intelligence, awareness and wellness begin at home.

A WORKBOOK FOR KIDS

Sometimes children can be overwhelmed by their emotions and not know how to deal with them.

The Kids' Workbook I have written can accompany this book and can be used in many ways:

- For a child to use on their own and not shared unless they want to. Treat it like a diary and allow the child some privacy.
- With a parent or caring adult in whose wisdom the child trusts to share their innermost thoughts.
- In a group or even a classroom where pages can be used at random when the opportunity arises.

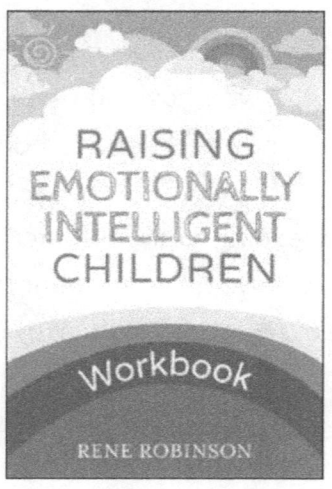

Use this book as a tool to help children think about how and what they are feeling, make it a bit of fun and remember not to judge.

I hope you find it useful and easy to use as this is my passion.

ON CHILDREN

KAHLIL GIBRAN - 1883-1931

And a woman who held a babe against her bosom said, Speak to us of Children.
    And he said:
    Your children are not your children.
    They are the sons and daughters of Life's longing for itself.
    They come through you but not from you,
    And though they are with you yet they belong not to you.

    You may give them your love but not your thoughts,
    For they have their own thoughts.
    You may house their bodies but not their souls,
    For their souls dwell in the house of tomorrow, which you cannot visit, not even in your dreams.
    You may strive to be like them, but seek not to make them like you.
    For life goes not backward nor tarries with yesterday.
    You are the bows from which your children as living arrows are sent forth.
    The archer sees the mark upon the path of the infinite, and He bends you with His might that His arrows may go swift and far.
    Let your bending in the archer's hand be for gladness;
    For even as He loves the arrow that flies, so He loves also the bow that is stable.

The Prophet[4]

ACKNOWLEDGEMENTS

As I have been fortunate to have learnt from some of the greatest teachers throughout my journey, I would like to acknowledge them here:

My parents, my sibling family and my extended family who helped me to shape and live my life, presented me with opportunities to grow and to experience life. Wonderful parents who gave me all the opportunities they were able to provide, including music tuition, especially important for me, sewing and an education which helped me to develop and follow my love of learning.

Various school teachers who encouraged this outgoing lass to open her mind.

My three sons – Luke, Mitch and Nick, who lived their childhood with this cranky schoolteacher mum and survived to become caring, independent adult men and fathers.

My first two granddaughters, Dakota and Summer, who came to live with me as little people and stayed for twenty years. This relationship and years of sharing my life with the girls has added to the depth of my story. All of the work we did together paid off as Dakota and Summer are now successful young adults, working and living independently, emotionally well and wise.

As life as a kinship carer became emotionally harder for me, I asked for help from my local GP and friend, Doctor Jo (Andrew) Horwood. Jo became one of the greatest links in the chain of my existence as he supported me and introduced me to special people able to help me on my journey, as well as supporting me too. I have the deepest gratitude for Jo as his was the first hand to be held out to me. He accepted me and challenged my enquiring mind.

Jo led me to Nicholas de Castella, who was the founder of 'The Institute of Heart Intelligence' in Melbourne. Nicholas ran 'Passionately Alive' workshops and through these I was able to access my anger and learn to let it go safely. I followed through Nicholas's courses and attained my 'Breathwork Therapist's' accreditation. I also used his work as a basis for my own work with children.

Thank you too to Susan and Cathy de Castella, who were also part of this great learning.

Thanks to the people behind 'The Journey' program – Brandon Bays, Kevin Billett, and all of the wonderful teachers, trainers and participants I was blessed to meet and learn from. This is truly the most powerful modality of healing I have learned and used in my work with children.

Thanks to Kevin and Kim Dallinger who made it possible for me to meet so many of my clients through their work at Villa Maria / Villa Maria Catholic Homes.

Thanks to my clients who trusted me and shared their lives and feelings with me. You all helped me grow and develop the skills I learned to use.

Thank you to the team at Dean Publishing for their work in developing this book and supporting this tardy writer.

ABOUT THE AUTHOR

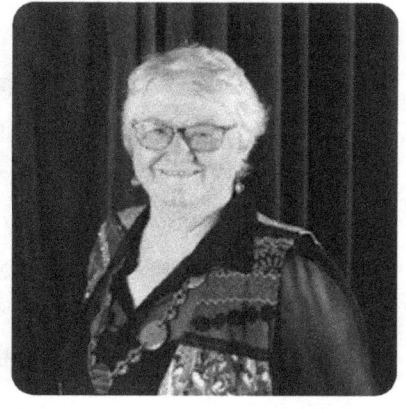

Rene has worn many hats and fulfilled many roles over the years. She has been a daughter, sister, friend, wife, teacher, single parent, grandparent, counsellor, traveller and so much more.

Children have always been Rene's passion, so teaching primary age children gave her the chance to develop her own interest in how children develop. Once she began her own work in emotional wellness, this passion grew and became her life's work.

Rene realised she could adapt this learning and make it easy for children to learn about their emotions and how to deal with them. From her work with her students, her clients and her granddaughters her original book was born, and from there this revised book and a corresponding Children's Workbook have been published.

Rene is a qualified primary school teacher with many years of experience. She has also worked as a school librarian, a hotel/motel publican, a counsellor, reiki master, teacher of tai chi, breathwork therapist and Journey practitioner.

Rene's love of travel has seen her travel to China to learn tai chi and, returning again in 1998, to teach English.

At the age of fifty-six and looking forward to her retirement, as well as further travel, Rene became full time carer to her two infant granddaughters, ten months and two years old at the time.

Determined not to see her granddaughters go into foster care, Rene took the two little girls into her home, and reared them for the next twenty years.

During this time, Rene also trained as an emotional wellness counsellor and worked for the 'Carers Network', co-facilitating sessions for support staff and providers. This led to her conducting one-to-one sessions with clients all over western Victoria.

In 2016, Rene re-visited Nepal as she had become involved in making and supplying sanitary kits for local girls in need. The goal of this trip was not only to supply the kits, but also to teach the girls in outlying and mountainous villages how to sew their own. It was a very successful trip and reinforced her love for Nepal.

She organised for a group to travel to Kathmandu and the Gorkha valley at the end of March 2020, to deliver sanitary supplies to other villages, when COVID struck. She hopes to return to Nepal soon to continue.

Thanks to the rich life she continues to lead, Rene is a sought-after speaker at Probus and Rotary meetings.

Rene's commitment to teaching people about emotional wellness remains strong and she continues to further her learning through experience and courses that answer this need.

According to Rene you are never too old to learn, and you are never too young to learn about understanding your emotions.

www.emotionalwellnessforkids.com.au

ENDNOTES

1. Dr Jo Horwood was my GP for many years. Dr Horwood's article 'How Shames Makes Us Sick' cannot be currently sourced online however I would like to acknowledge the impact it had on my work and personal life.
2. DeCastella, Nicholas. 'The Anatomy of Shame' [online article] - retrieved 23 rd August 2021. http://www.eq.net.au/wp-content/themes/emotional/pdf% 27s/AnatomyofShame.pdf
3. Gibran, Kahlil. *The Prophet*. Pocket ed. New York: Knopf, 1995.
4. Gibran, Kahlil. *The Prophet*, Knopf, 1923 , New York. (Public domain).

CPSIA information can be obtained
at www.ICGtesting.com
Printed in the USA
BVHW081953151221
624018BV00005B/668